Practical Ultrasound:
An Illustrated Guide

Dedicated to the memory of
Dr Donal Deery

Practical Ultrasound:
An Illustrated Guide

Jane Alty MB BChir MA MRCP
Specialist Registrar,
St James's University Hospital, Leeds, UK

Edward Hoey MB BCh BAO MRCP
Specialist Registrar,
St James's University Hospital, Leeds, UK

With collaboration from
Stephen Wolstenhulme MHSc DMU and
Michael Weston MB ChB MRCP FRCR

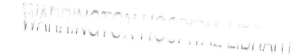

The ROYAL
SOCIETY *of*
MEDICINE
PRESS *Limited*

© 2006 Royal Society of Medicine Press Ltd

Published by the Royal Society of Medicine Press Ltd
1 Wimpole Street, London W1G 0AE, UK
Tel: +44 (0)20 7290 2921
Fax: +44 (0)20 7290 2929
Email: publishing@rsm.ac.uk
Website: www.rsmpress.co.uk

British Library Cataloguing in Publication Data
A catalogue record for this book is available from the British Library

ISBN 1-85315-603-5

Distribution in Europe and Rest of World:

Marston Book Services Ltd
PO Box 269
Abingdon
Oxon OX14 4YN, UK
Tel: +44 (0)1235 465500
Fax: +44 (0)1235 465555
Email: direct.order@marston.co.uk

Distribution in the USA and Canada:

Royal Society of Medicine Press Ltd
c/o BookMasters Inc
30 Amberwood Parkway
Ashland, OH 44805, USA
Tel: +1 800 247 6553/+1 800 266 5564
Fax: +1 419 281 6883
Email: order@bookmasters.com

Distribution in Australia and New Zealand:

Elsevier Australia
30–52 Smidmore Street
Marrikville NSW 2204, Australia
Tel: +61 2 9517 8999
Fax: +61 2 9517 2249
Email: service@elsevier.com.au

Designed and typeset by Phoenix Photosetting, Chatham, Kent

Printed in the Netherlands by Alfabase, Alphen aan den Rijn

Contents

Foreword

In the hands of a properly trained operator, ultrasound scanning seems simple, just slide the probe over the body surface and beautiful images of the body's interior appear on the screen. The skilled operator will point out the detailed anatomy and pathological features, as if it were effortless. But there lies the rub – it can be an illusion. As has been so often pointed out, the problem with ultrasound is that it is totally operator dependant and skilled operators need to be properly trained; and, after 30 years' experience, I can report that the training in ultrasound of sonographers, radiologists, and other medical and surgical specialists can be a long and tedious business!

But, help has now arrived. This book will ease the pain and will undoubtedly assist the beginner to learn how to operate the equipment, how to scan, and how to interpret what appears on the screen. It has been written by two recent radiology trainees (Jane Alty and Edward Hoey) who, whilst going through that initial learning phase, realised that a practical manual such as this would greatly assist the learning process. They have collaborated with two experienced ultrasound trainers. Stephen Wolstenhulme, a sonographer, is an invaluable member of the Radiology Department at St James's University Hospital, who has endless patience and has spent countless hours helping trainee sonographers and radiologists through those vital first steps of learning to image with ultrasound; and Michael Weston, a consultant radiologist colleague who supported the idea from the beginning and provided much encouragement and help throughout the project.

The authors are to be congratulated for their efforts. They have seen an obvious need and, based on their own experience, have provided the solution. This book will be of tremendous value to all who are learning to use ultrasound, whether they are sonographers, radiologists, or other medical and surgical specialists who are following the recently published guidance from the Royal College of Radiologists, *Ultrasound Training Recommendations for Medical and Surgical Specialties*, 2005.

If you are reading this Foreword prior to embarking on an ultrasound training programme, then you are indeed fortunate. Not only are you on the brink of discovering a wonderful world of non-invasive imaging, but also your pathway to achieving the competence that you desire will be made considerably easier by this book.

Henry C Irving FRCR
Consultant Radiologist
St James's University Hospital, Leeds, UK;
Ex-Treasurer of The Royal College of Radiologists

Preface

If this is your first exposure to clinical ultrasound then understandably you may feel a little overwhelmed right now – but don't worry, this book has been written with precisely you in mind. It was put together during our first ultrasound placement as registrars on the St James's University Hospital, Leeds radiology scheme, so we know how you feel in this unfamiliar territory.

The aim of this book is to help you learn how to scan. This book will take you through all the common scans that you will encounter in a busy ultrasound department. The chapters are organized according to anatomical sites. Each chapter comprises a revision section on useful anatomy, a scan protocol presented in a step-by-step approach, and a section on common pathology. We have kept things as simple as possible without going into the detailed physics that underlies ultrasound scanning. Although the approach is simple, the volume of knowledge you will attain while learning to scan is immense. We hope that the skills you learn through using this book will be the foundation upon which you can build up your knowledge in the future.

We recommend that you start by reading the relevant chapter prior to scanning and then attempt to follow the steps that you have read about. It may be useful to have the book beside you as you scan as a quick reference. Once you master the basics, you will find yourself needing to refer less to the instructions column, and you simply follow the scan steps to ensure that all the necessary areas are covered.

In each chapter, we have included some examples of both common and clinically relevant pathologies, as well as some notes on the salient features of these conditions. We have not provided an exhaustive list of pathologies, but instead have highlighted the common ones to look out for while learning to scan.

Jane Alty
Edward Hoey
Stephen Wolstenhulme
Michael Weston

Abbreviations

AA	arch of the aorta		IUCD	intrauterine contraceptive device
AAL	anterior axillary line		IVC	inferior vena cava
ACA	anterior cerebral artery		IVDU	intravenous drug use
Ao	aorta		LHV	left hepatic vein
AP	anteroposterior		LIF	left iliac fossa
AT	acceleration time		LMP	last menstrual period
BCA	brachiocephalic artery		LPV	left portal vein
β-hCG	β human chorionic gonadotrophin		LRA	left renal artery
BPD	biparietal diameter		LRV	left renal vein
CBD	common bile duct		LS	longitudinal section
CCA	common carotid artery		LSC	left subclavian artery
CCF	congestive cardiac failure		LSV	long saphenous vein
CF	cystic fibrosis		LUQ	left upper quadrant
CIA	common iliac artery		MCA	middle cerebral artery
COPD	chronic obstructive pulmonary disease		MCL	midclavicular line
CRF	chronic renal failure		MHA	main hepatic artery
CRL	crown–rump length		MHV	middle hepatic vein
D	end-diastole		MHz	megaHertz
DVT	deep vein thrombosis		MI	mechanical index
EBV	Epstein–Barr virus		MPV	main portal vein
ECA	external carotid artery		MRA	main renal artery
ECG	electrocardiogram		MRI	magnetic resonance imaging
EDF	end-diastolic flow		MSD	mean sac diameter
EDV	end-diastolic velocity		MRV	main renal vein
EIA	external iliac artery		OA	osteoarthritis
ERCP	endoscopic retrograde cholangiopancreatography		OCP	oral contraceptive pill
			PACS	patient archive communication system
FOV	field of view		PBC	primary biliary cirrhosis
GB	gallbladder		PCA	posterior cerebral artery
HA	hepatic artery		PCKD	polycystic kidney disease
HAT	hepatic artery thrombosis		PCOS	polycystic ovarian syndrome
HCC	hepatocellular carcinoma		PN	pyelonephritis
HRT	hormone replacement therapy		PLiSK	'pancreas, liver, spleen, kidneys' (see Chapter 1, point 7)
HV	hepatic vein			
ICA	internal carotid artery		PRF	pulse repetition frequency
ICS	intercostal space		PSC	primary sclerosing cholangitis
ICU	intensive care unit		PSV	peak-systolic velocity
IHD	ischaemic heart disease		PTLD	post-transplant lymphoproliferative disorder
IHF	interhemispheric fissure			
IIA	internal iliac artery		PV	portal vein
IJV	internal jugular vein		RA	right atrium
IMA	inferior mesenteric artery		RAS	renal artery stenosis

RCC	renal cell carcinoma		SCM	sternocleidomastoid muscle
RHA	right hepatic artery		SMA	superior mesenteric artery
RHV	right hepatic vein		SMV	superior mesenteric vein
RI	resistance index		SNR	signal-to-noise ratio
RIF	right iliac fossa		SSV	short saphenous vein
RPOC	retained products of conception		SV	splenic vein
RPV	right portal vein		SVC	superior vena cava
RRA	right renal artery		TA	transabdominal
RRV	right renal vein		TCC	transitional cell carcinoma
RSC	right subclavian artery		TGC	time gain control
RSI	repetitive strain injury		TS	transverse section
RUQ	right upper quadrant		TV	tricuspid valve; transvaginal
RV	right ventricle		WRULD	work-related upper-limb disorder

Acknowledgements

We would like to thank our family and friends for their support during the writing of this book. We are especially indebted to Dr Carsten Grimm for designing several of the probe position diagrams and for his technical computer wizardry throughout the text. We are most grateful to the ultrasonographers of St James's University Hospital and Seacroft Hospital for their teaching, guidance and patience, namely Mr Ian Entwistle, Ms Pat Duffin, Ms Orlaigh McGuiness, Mr Roger Lapham, Mr Mike Kirk, Mrs Debbie Carr and Mrs Alison Mackintosh. Finally, we would like to acknowledge the staff of the medical illustration department at St James's University Hospital for their kind assistance in editing our collected images, and to Dr Richard Fowler, Dr Chirag Patel, Ms Linda Arundale and Ms Joanne Leivars for providing key images that have added immensely to the quality of this book.

Table of values

System/organ	Structure/measurement	Normal size/range
Abdomen	Gallbladder wall thickness	<3 mm
	Pancreatic duct	<2 mm
	CBD diameter	<6 mm
	CBD diameter (postcholecystectomy)	<9 mm
	IVC AP diameter	<2 cm
	Spleen length	<13 cm
	Portal vein flow	10–20 cm/s
Abdominal aorta	Aorta AP diameter	<2 cm
	CIA AP diameter	<1 cm
Carotids	0–49% stenosis	<1.5 m/s
	50–69% stenosis	1.5–2.3 m/s
	>70% stenosis	>2.3 m/s
Gynaecological	Ovarian volume	<10 cm^3
	Endometrial thickness:	
	• premenopausal	<15 mm
	• postmenopausal	<5 mm
	Simple ovarian cyst diameter	<30 mm
	PCOS ovarian volume	>10 cm^3
Renal	Renal length LS	9–12 cm
	Renal cortical thickness	1.5–2.5 cm
	Residual bladder volume postmicturition	<100 cm^3
	Bladder wall thickness (distended)	<5 mm
	Resistance index	<0.7
	Normal ILA acceleration time	<0.07 s
	Renal artery stenosis (70%) acceleration time	>0.12 s
	Velocity in RAS measured directly from MRA:	
	• in native kidney	<1.8 m/s
	• in transplant kidney	<2.5 m/s
Testes	Testicular volume	>10 cm^3
Thyroid	Thyroid craniocaudal length in LS	<4 cm
	Normal thyroid nodule	<7 mm
	Parathyroid craniocaudal length in LS	<6 mm

1

General principles of ultrasound scanning

Here are some suggestions to help improve the quality of ultrasound scans and so increase the information obtained from them. There is also some advice on how to prevent repetitive strain injury (RSI)/work-related upper-limb disorder (WRULD)

1. Ensure correct orientation of the probe head to obtain conventional scan images. One designated end (marked on some probes with a ridge or light) should point towards the patient's head when scanning in the LS (longitudinal/coronal) plane, then, on turning 90° anticlockwise into a TS (transverse/axial) plane, this end will be pointing towards the patient's right side.

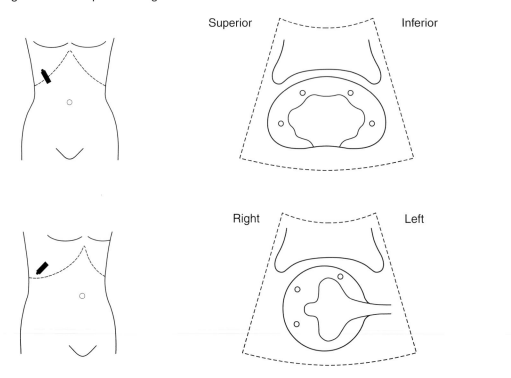

Hint: Running a finger along the probe face will produce a faint ripple on the screen, and it will be obvious which is the correct way round!

2. To avoid missing pathology at the peripheries of an organ, always scan completely off structures – e.g., for kidneys, scan completely through and beyond in both LS and TS planes.

3. To improve images, try to scan through an acoustic window whenever possible – e.g. through a full bladder for transabdominal pelvic scans.

4. When examining a cystic lesion, look for features to help characterize it as benign (e.g. a simple cyst) or potentially malignant:

Benign features:
- smooth edge
- thin wall
- echo-free contents
- postacoustic enhancement

Malignant features:
- irregular edge
- thick wall
- internal echoes/thick septations
- poor beam through transmission
- internal blood flow

5. Ultrasound is commonly used to look for malignant lesions, both within organs and in the adjacent tissues. Often the changes can be subtle, especially if the lesion is of a similar echogenicity to the surrounding tissue. One clue is to look for a 'mass effect', which is commonly seen with malignant tumours, whereby they cause distortion of the normal anatomical architecture – e.g. liver metastases often distort the hepatic and portal venous anatomy.

6. Make use of colour Doppler to help distinguish vessels from other structures – e.g. common bile duct versus portal vein/hepatic artery.

7. Use the mnemonic 'PLiSK' when comparing the echogenicity of the abdominal organs. The pancreas is normally a little more echo-bright than the liver, which in turn is normally slightly brighter than the spleen, which is brighter than the kidneys. PLiSK is a quick and easy way of remembering the correct sequence and will alert you to the presence of some pathologies – e.g. fatty liver, which appears much brighter than it should (see later).

P Li S K

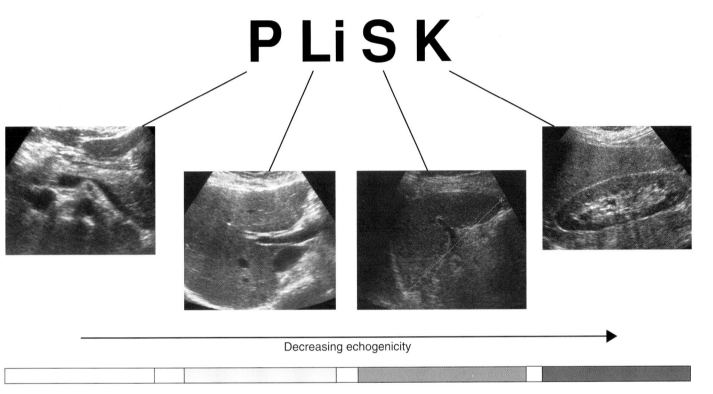

Decreasing echogenicity

8. When measuring blood vessel calibre, do so in TS with the probe perpendicular to the vessel; measure from inside of wall to inside of wall. This gives more reproducible measurements than in LS, when you are more likely to image a vessel in oblique section.

9. If bowel gas is obscuring a structure (e.g. the pancreas), try manoeuvres to move it out of the way – e.g. instruct the patient to 'push out stomach' or re-examine later after moving the patient. If the patient is not 'nil by mouth' then giving a waterload to fill the stomach to act as an acoustic window can also help to visualize midline structures.

10. When viewing abnormalities in a fluid-filled structure (e.g. gallstones), always try to obtain images after the patient has changed position. This will help distinguish lesions fixed to a wall (e.g. polyps) from mobile ones (e.g. stones). This also enables discrimination of stones from bowel gas and off-axis/slice thickness artefacts.

11. Always have consideration for patient safety. The mechanical index (MI), which is a measure of tissue effects from ultrasound, should always be kept to the lowest level that allows an image to be achieved. This is especially true when imaging sensitive structures such as the developing embryo. Regulations allow MIs up to a maximum of 0.9.

PREVENTING RSI/WRULD

This is a common problem among healthcare professionals who use ultrasound on a regular basis. It most often affects the upper limb of the scan arm and is thought to be caused by a combination of awkward posture due to poor workstation set-up and sustained static forces due to excessive twisting and pressure on the probe. The following measures will help to alleviate this problem:

• Try to have a mixed caseload during the scan session.
• Adjust the bed height in order to avoid stretching excessively up or down during the scan – have your eyes level with the top of the monitor to avoid excessive neck movements.
• Try to maintain good posture while seated for the scan – ergonomically designed stools can help with this.

- Try to rest the elbow of your scan arm gently on the patient.
- Keep close to the patient in order to avoid the need to abduct your arm excessively during the scan.
- Position the console so that it is not necessary to stretch excessively over the patient.
- Move the patient into oblique/decubitus positions when examining the kidneys/spleen. This prevents excessive rotation of the forearm.
- Apply only light skin pressure with the probe.
- Remember to stretch and to take regular rest periods between patients.

2

Guide to using the ultrasound machine

1. Confirm the patient's name, date of birth and address.
2. Reassure the patient as to the nature of the examination.
3. Enter the patient's details into the machine (usually via a 'patient data button'). If using a PACS system, use the worklist to select the patient.
4. Select the transducer:
   - abdomen/renal/transabdominal gynaecological scans: curvilinear broad-bandwidth probe with low central frequency (3–5 MHz)
   - transvaginal gynaecological scans: endovaginal broad-bandwidth probe with high central frequency (5–8 MHz)
   - testis/thyroid/vascular scans: linear broad-bandwidth probe with high central frequency (6–10 MHz) (select the highest frequency that allows penetration through the structure)
5. Select the application or 'preset' (the body part that is to be scanned). The machine then adjusts its postprocessing algorithm accordingly – e.g. 'carotid' will increase edge definition and contrast and decrease frame averaging.
6. If using a laser-print storage system, enter the patient's details (e.g. patient ID number).
7. Adjust the ambient light levels in the room.
8. Apply an aqueous gel (which acts as a coupling medium) to the scan area.
9. Proceed to scan using the guidelines outlined in this book.
10. Optimize the image quality using the following functions:
    (a) **Depth**. Increase or decrease this so that the area of interest fills the screen.
    (b) **Overall gain**. Turning this up or down will adjust the overall image 'brightness'.
    (c) **Focus**. Place the focus position (indicated by a small marker on the side of the screen) to the bottom of the area of interest. By selecting two or three 'focal zones', the lateral resolution of the scan can be improved (e.g. good for testis or TS kidney); however, the trade-off is a slower frame rate (slower image update).

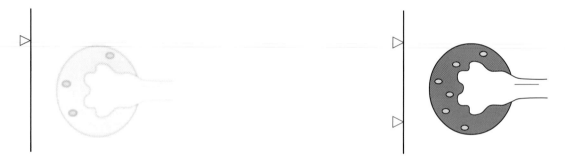

One focal zone – not set deep enough

Two focal zones set correctly

    (d) **Time gain control (TGC)**. This works by amplifying weak returning echoes from varying depths. It increases or decreases brightness at these levels. Start with the TGC in a vertical line in the middle of the scale and adjust from here – e.g., for bladder imaging, it can be adjusted to remove anterior wall reverberation artefacts:

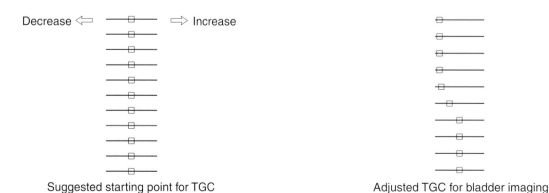

Decrease ⇐ ⇒ Increase

Suggested starting point for TGC

Adjusted TGC for bladder imaging

    (e) **Field of view (FOV)**. By reducing this to the smallest required area, the frame rate will be maximized, which increases the line density and thus improves image resolution:

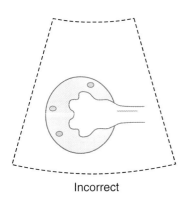
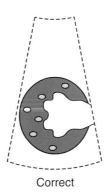

| Incorrect | Correct |

(f) Frequency. With a multifrequency transducer, the following options are available:

(i) Increase the frequency for viewing superficial structures/thin patients. This will improve resolution.

(ii) Reduce the frequency for viewing deeper structures/large patients in order to improve penetration.

(g) Resolution/speed. On some machines, this can be adjusted. The scale ranges from 1 to 5, and by setting it at 4 or 5, the detail in the image will be improved – but at the expense of a reduced frame rate, e.g.

resolution/speed of 1 = 17 frames/s image update

resolution/speed of 5 = 10 frames/s image update

(h) Tissue harmonics. This generally sharpens up the image by reducing signal from the fat layers and improving edge definition (it is known as the registrar button!). However, it slows the frame rate, and on some machines it significantly decreases the penetration. For certain body parts, especially superficial structures, it is not advised.

(i) Zoom. This magnifies the screen image, which is useful for viewing small structures like ovaries. It can be used during dynamic scanning or when the image is frozen. It has no effect on the frame rate.

(j) Parallel. This function is available on some machines. It improves resolution by sending out two signals side by side, which increases the frame rate and allows the use of multiple focal zones, which in turn improves the resolution. If this function is available, most operators use it all the time.

(k) Acoustic (output) power. If overall gain and TGC are at maximum and it is still not possible to penetrate a structure (e.g. the liver) at the desired frequency, then try to increase this. However, safety must be considered, and the mechanical index (MI) should always be kept to the lowest level that allows an image to be obtained.

(l) Doppler functions. Doppler ultrasound gives blood flow information. There are several different ways in which it can be utilized:

(i) *Colour Doppler*. When this is selected, a 'box' appears and a colour map of flow within vessels in this region of interest is displayed. The colours used are usually red and blue to indicate flow towards and away from the probe respectively – but the operator can adjust this.

(ii) *Power Doppler*. This is similar to colour Doppler in that blood flow is displayed over a region of interest; however, no directional information is given. It is more sensitive for detecting low-velocity flow, as it summates the signal from all the frequency shifts.

(iii) *Spectral Doppler*. When this is selected, a 'gate marker' appears, which the operator places over the vessel of interest. This then gives detailed analysis of flow velocities at this one site, displaying them as a waveform above and below the baseline to indicate flow towards and away from the probe respectively – the operator can reverse this if desired by selecting the 'spectral invert' function. The spectral Doppler trace can usually be displayed on screen alongside either a 'frozen' scan image or the 'real-time' image. The real-time image will have a slower frame rate than a regular colour image, but it can still be useful when trying to locate small vessels that are moving with respiration (e.g. renal interlobar arteries). In practice, most operators adjust between the two.

Optimizing colour Doppler

1. First select a probe that gives adequate penetration through to the region of interest. If flow cannot be seen, consider changing to a lower-frequency probe (better penetration).

2. Ensure that the 'preset' (see above) is correct for the area being examined, as the machine adjusts the colour set-up and colour processing algorithm according to this.

3. Place the focus position at the level of the vessels of interest and reduce the size of the colour box to cover only this area.

4. If the colour signal is weak, try increasing the colour gain and reducing the overall sector width.

5. Adjust the scale/pulse repetition frequency (PRF). This controls how frequently pulses are sent from the probe to detect flow:
   - for slow moving blood (e.g. venous), select low scale/PRF
   - for fast moving blood (e.g. arterial), select high scale/PRF

   If the scale/PRF is set incorrectly, aliasing may occur where high velocities get misregistered, resulting in wrapping around of the waveform, or there can be a loss of sensitivity to low velocities.

6. Adjust the filter settings for what is required. The filter can be set to cut out all signals below a certain frequency shift (this is good for removing noise). However, when trying to detect low flow velocities, the position of the baseline needs to be adjusted to a lower level or the filter turned off altogether – e.g. in cases of suspected testicular torsion.

7. Adjust the probe position/angle-correct function until the angle between the beam and the vessel of interest is between 0° and 60° (see below).

Optimizing power Doppler. All of the above points apply, but as no velocity or directional flow is being measured, points 5 and 7 are not as important.

Optimizing spectral Doppler. The points listed above for colour Doppler are all important. In addition, to ensure accurate estimation of the flow velocity:

1. Ensure that the beam-flow angle is between 0° and 60°, because if the vessel is running at or near right-angles, calculated velocities are unreliable (as cos 90° = 0). Adjust the angle via:
   - positioning of probe
   - angle-correct function

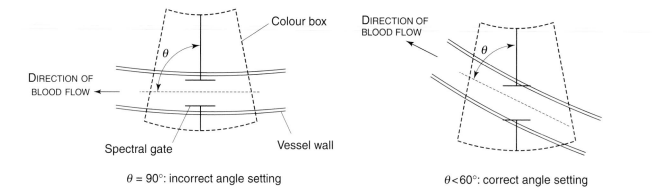

$\theta = 90°$: incorrect angle setting $\theta < 60°$: correct angle setting

Hint: When using a linear probe (e.g. when imaging leg veins or carotids), it is important to steer the colour box along the direction of flow in the vessel. Again aim for a beam-flow angle < 60° for accurate velocity calculations:

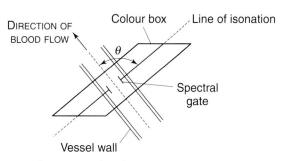   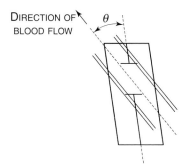

Incorrect colour box steer: $\theta > 60°$.   Correct colour box steer: $\theta < 60°$.
This will cause overestimation of flow velocity   This allows accurate estimation of flow velocity

2. The gate size (sample volume) should be adjusted to fill the whole vessel – e.g. if it is too big then signals from nearby vessels may be included:

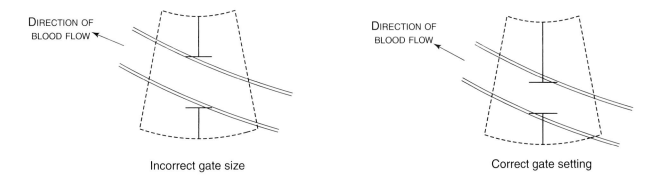

Incorrect gate size   Correct gate setting

(m) M-mode function. When this is selected, a line appears, which the operator places across the site of interest. The display then shows only the echoes from this one line, but plotted against time. This reveals movement of structures towards and away from the probe. It is used in early pregnancy scanning (see Chapter 10).

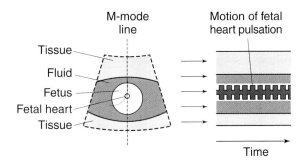

When the images appear to be satisfactory, start recording them:

11. Press the freeze button to get a still image.
12. Some systems allow review of the last few seconds before this via a 'ciné loop'.
13. Distances can be marked via the measurement function and tracker ball.
14. It is good practice to label images via either bodymarkers or typescript.
15. Once the examination is complete, end study on the machine and store/print images according to the set-up in the department – e.g. PACS, Hardcopy, etc.

3
Abdomen

USEFUL ABDOMINAL ANATOMY

Try not be too daunted by the complexity of the abdominal anatomy. It is not necessary to learn every branch of every artery and every relationship of every organ at once – start by learning the basics well and then build up more detailed knowledge on this foundation. Here we summarize three TS sections at important vertebral levels and three useful LS sections. Learn the important points from these schematic diagrams and then through scanning experience, create a mental picture of the three-dimensional structure of the abdominal contents and their key relationships. When scanning, one should look out for the key anatomical points listed below. Over time, with the acquisition of anatomical knowledge, you will begin to develop pattern recognition for what is normal and what is not.

TS: T12 level
Probe position
(immediately inferior to xiphisternum)

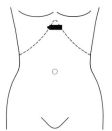

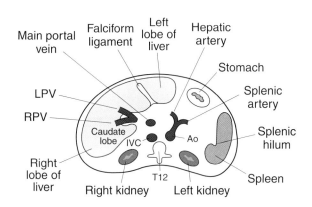

Key points

1. The coeliac axis arises from the aorta at the T12 level.
2. The coeliac axis branches into the splenic artery and the hepatic artery – this branching appears as a 'seagull' shape when seen in TS.
3. The falciform ligament separates the liver into anatomical left and right lobes.
4. The splenic vein and superior mesenteric vein join to form the portal vein at T12/L1.
5. The portal vein branches into the right and left portal veins at the porta hepatis.

TS: L1 level
Probe position
(halfway between xiphisterum
and umbilicus)

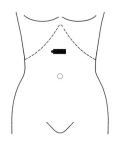

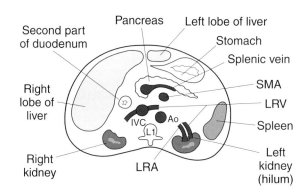

Key points

1. The left renal hilum lies approximately 2 cm more superiorly than the right renal hilum.
2. The left renal vein passes anterior to the aorta.
3. The right renal artery passes posterior to the inferior vena cava.
4. The pancreas lies immediately anterior to the splenic vein.
5. The splenic vein is 'tadpole'-shaped when imaged in TS – i.e. the 'head' of the tadpole is the portal confluence and the 'tail' is the splenic vein.

TS: L2 level
Probe position
(just superior to umbilicus)

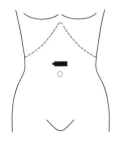

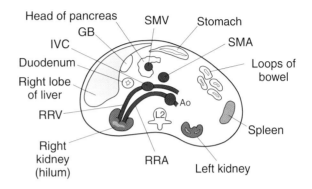

Key points

1. The renal arteries branch off the aorta at L2.
2. The renal veins lie anterior to the renal arteries.
3. The superior mesenteric vein and splenic vein join to form the portal vein posterior to the neck of the pancreas.
4. The aorta bifurcates just inferior to this level at L3/4.

LS: right MCL
Probe position

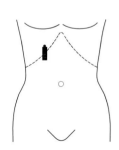

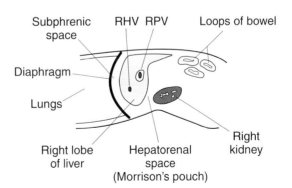

LS: right of midline
Probe position

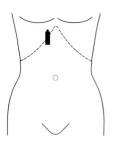

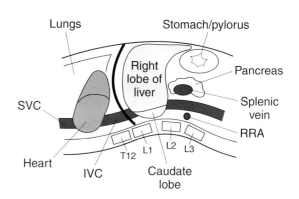

LS: left of midline
Probe position

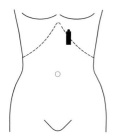

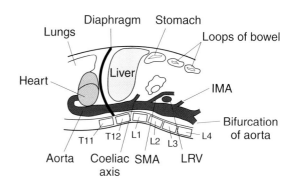

PERITONEAL SPACES

TS
Probe position: L1

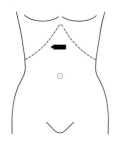

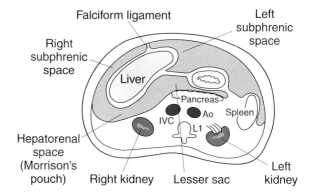

LS
Probe position: right MCL

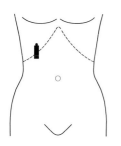

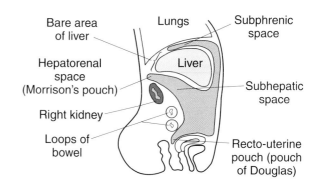

Key points

1. The spaces are formed between folds of peritoneum.
2. These spaces are where free fluid accumulates.
3. Morrison's pouch is the most dependent part of the abdominal cavity when the patient is supine. Therefore ALWAYS examine here for free fluid.

ANATOMY OF THE PORTA HEPATIS AND BILIARY SYSTEM

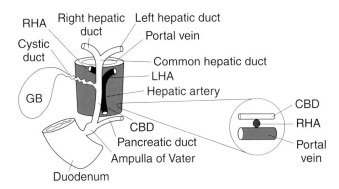

Key points

1. The right hepatic artery runs between the common bile duct and portal vein in 90% of patients.
2. The right and left hepatic ducts join at the porta hepatis to form the common hepatic duct.
3. The common hepatic duct joins the cystic duct to form the common bile duct.
4. The common bile duct joins the pancreatic duct to form the ampulla of Vater, which empties into the duodenum.

SEGMENTS OF THE LIVER

Initially, it is acceptable to describe the position of abnormalities as either in the left or right lobe:

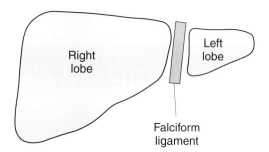

Eventually, however, it is worth learning the surgical segments of the liver in order to describe any abnormalities more accurately:

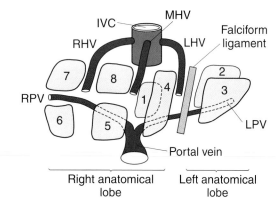

Viewed from above, the appearance is as follows:

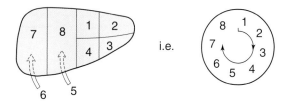

i.e.

Key points

1. The liver is divided into eight surgical segments by the branches of the portal and hepatic veins as shown above.
2. When viewed from above, the segments are numbered clockwise 1–8.
3. Segment 1 is the caudate lobe.
4. Segment 4 is a good place to look for focal fatty sparing or focal fatty infiltration.
5. Segment 6 extends beyond the inferior border of the right kidney in hepatomegaly.
6. 75% of the liver's native blood supply is from the portal vein and 25% is from the hepatic artery.
7. The liver is drained via the three hepatic veins into the inferior vena cava.
8. Intrahepatic portal veins have echo-bright walls.

ECHOGENICITY OF ABDOMINAL ORGANS

Remember the mnemonic PLiSK when comparing the echogenicity of the abdominal organs (see Chapter 1):

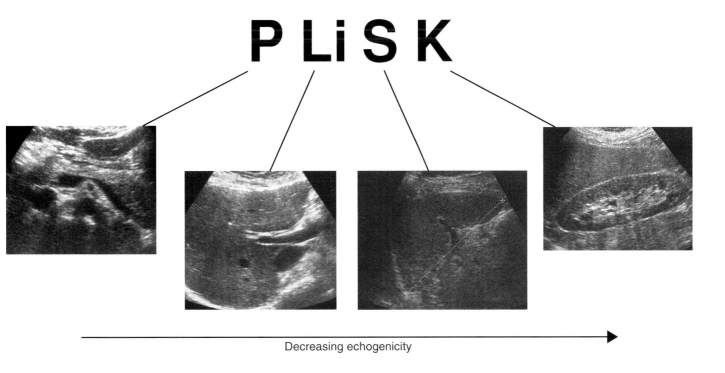

Decreasing echogenicity

PERFORMING THE SCAN

- **Patient position**: Supine.
- **Preparation**: Nil by mouth or just clear fluids for 8 hours.
- **Probe**: Low-frequency (3–5 MHz) curvilinear.
- **Machine**: Select the abdomen preset mode. Use tissue harmonics if the SNR is poor or with obese patients.
- **Method**: Acquire more than just representative images for each step if pathology is found.

Probe position	*Instructions*

1. Midline – TS: pancreas
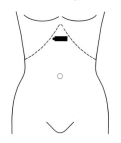
	• Place the probe perpendicular to the upper abdomen in the midline. Look for the 'tadpole' shape of the splenic vein (tail) and portal confluence (head), and then look anterior to this to locate the pancreas.
	• Scan through the whole pancreas by angling the probe cranially then caudally. Take note of the following pancreas characteristics:
	  – size: is it swollen (acute pancreatitis)?
	  – echogenicity (bright = fat infiltration)
	  – any masses/cysts?
	  – dilated pancreatic duct (>2 mm)?
	  – any calcifications (chronic pancreatitis)?
	• Acquire representative image(s).

2. Midline – LS: pancreas
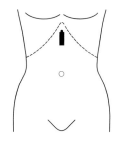
	• Turn the probe clockwise through 90° in order to scan in LS. Look for the splenic vein and then look anterior to this to locate the pancreas.
	• Scan through the whole pancreas by angling the probe laterally right and left.
	• If the pancreas cannot be found, try scanning:
	  – again at the end of the examination
	  – after filling the stomach with water
	  – with the patient in the lateral decubitus position to move overlying bowel out of the way
	  – with the patient sitting erect
	• Take note of the characteristics as listed in Step 1.
	• Acquire representative image(s).

3. Midline – TS: aorta 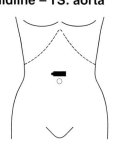	• Turn the probe anticlockwise through 90° in order to scan in TS again. • Increase the depth and look for the aorta. • Turn on colour Doppler if there is difficulty in finding the aorta (especially in obese patients). • Follow the course of the aorta down to the bifurcation, looking for any aneurysms or atherosclerosis. • Measure the AP diameter of the aorta at its widest point. • Acquire representative image(s).

What to look for

Scan image

1.

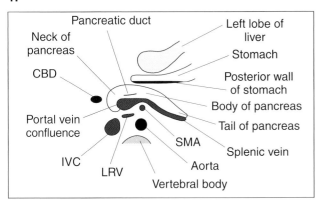

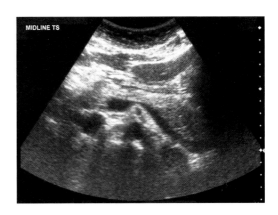

Tadpole head = portal vein confluence
Tadpole tail = splenic vein
Hint: Do not mistake the posterior wall of the stomach for a dilated pancreatic duct!

2.

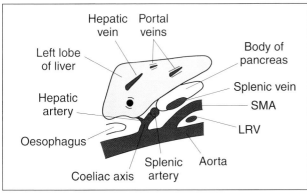

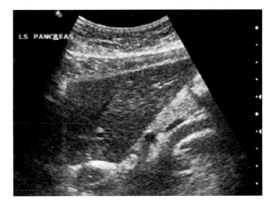

3.

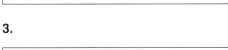

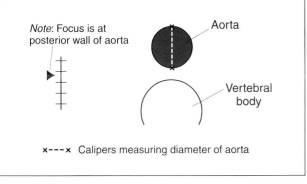

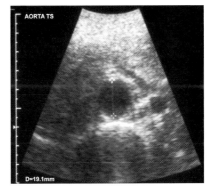

Probe position	**Instructions**

4. Midline – TS: left lobe of liver

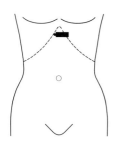

- Keep the probe TS and in the midline. Scan through the whole of the left lobe of the liver by angling the probe cranially then caudally.
- Take note of:
    - the echogenicity: diffuse and focal
    - the size
    - the surface: is it smooth or nodular, is it cirrhotic?
    - the bile ducts: are they dilated?
    - any lesions: do they have mass effect?
    - hepatic and portal veins
- If there is difficulty in viewing the liver clearly, ask the patient to take a deep breath in to push the liver down.
- Acquire representative image(s).

5. LS: aorta and left lobe of liver

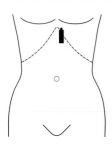

- Turn the probe clockwise through 90° into LS and place it just left of the midline.
- Increase the depth as necessary and look for the aorta in LS.
- Look specifically for the SMA branching off and passing over the LRV.
- Examine the left lobe of the liver by sweeping the probe towards the LUQ.
- Make sure to scan completely off the liver edge, as this is a common place for metastases to 'hide'.
- Take note of the liver characteristics listed in Step 4.
- Acquire representative image(s).

6. LS: IVC and caudate

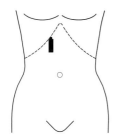

- Keep the probe in LS and move a little to the right of the midline.
- Look for the IVC passing through the liver with the caudate lobe anteriorly and posteriorly.
- Take note of the liver characteristics listed in Step 4.
- Examine the IVC for:
    - dilation with expiration (normal)
    - size (>2 cm AP diameter in CCF)
- Acquire representative image(s).

What to look for

Scan image

4.

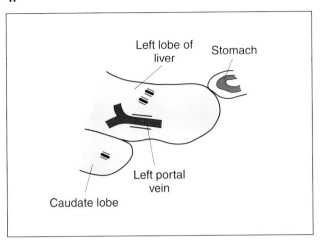

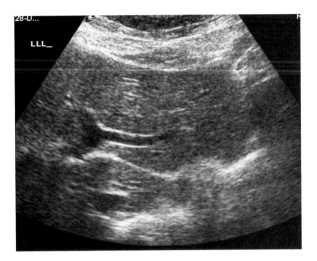

5.

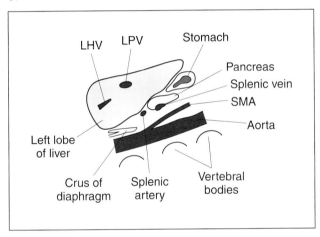

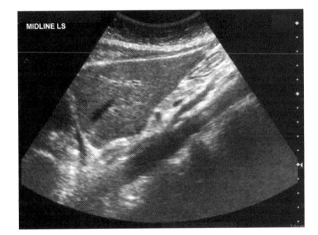

6.

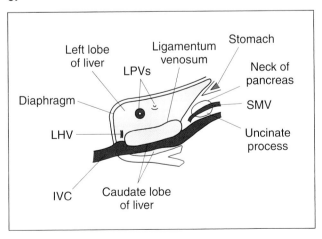

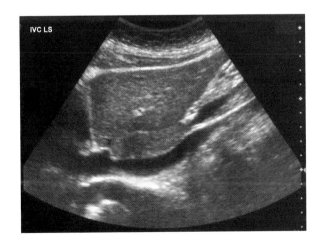

Probe position	**Instructions**

7. LS: porta hepatis and CBD measurement

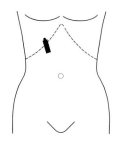

- Keep in LS and move the probe further to the patient's right.
- Take note of the liver characteristics listed in Step 4.
- Look for the portal vein and follow its course it into the liver. The porta hepatis is the region where the vein enters the liver. At this point, look for the CBD by rotating the probe slightly anticlockwise and looking anterior to the portal vein. The hepatic artery runs between the duct and the portal vein (usually).
- To help locate the CBD:
  - turn on colour: no flow in CBD
  - increase line density by reducing sector angle and depth
  - use zoom to magnify the area
- Follow the course of the CBD, looking for any calculi or obstruction.
- Measure the CBD at its widest point. It should be <6 mm (or <9 mm post-cholecystectomy).
- Remember to also look specifically for lymph nodes at the porta hepatis.
- Acquire representative image(s).

8. LS: right liver medial to right kidney

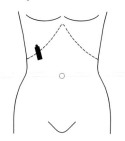

- Keep in LS and move the probe further to the patient's right. Sweep the probe laterally to the left and then right, examining the right lobe of the liver.
- Take note of the liver characteristics listed in Step 4.
- Remember to also look above and below the diaphragm for any pleural effusions/free fluid/subphrenic collections during this step.
- Acquire representative image(s).

9. LS: right kidney/liver

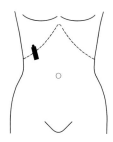

- Keep in LS and move the probe further to the right (usually MCL) to image the right kidney and the right lobe of the liver together.
- Sweep laterally towards the RUQ, examining the liver characteristics. Make sure to scan completely off the right edge of the liver.
- Compare the echogenicity of the liver parenchyma and renal cortex (liver should be a little brighter – remember PLiSK!).
- Look for hepatomegaly:
  - Does segment 6 of the liver extend below the inferior renal pole?
  - Is the angle of the liver >45°, i.e. rounded?
- Look for any fluid in the hepatorenal space (Morrison's pouch).
- Acquire representative image(s).

What to look for	*Scan image*

7.

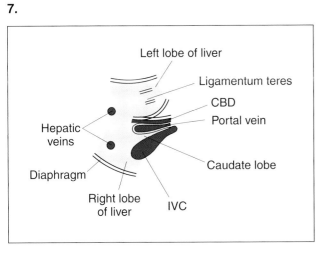

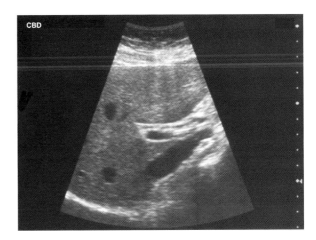

8.

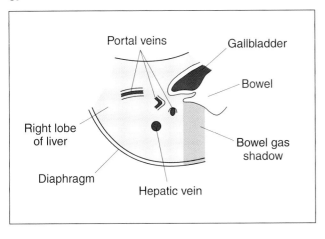

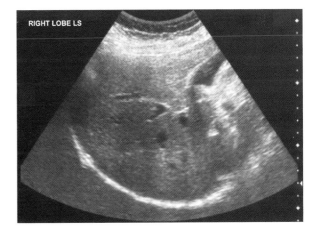

9.

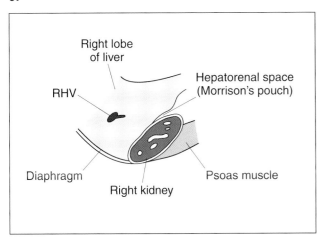

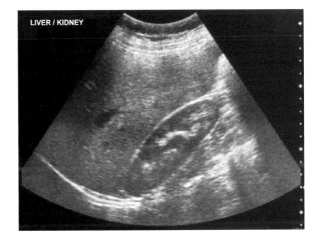

Remember the mnemonic PLiSK – i.e. the pancreas is normally the most echogenic organ, then the liver, then the spleen, then the kidney.

Probe position	**Instructions**

10. TS: liver – level of hepatic veins

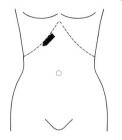

- Place the probe parallel and inferior to the right costal margin to scan the liver in TS.
- Ask the patient to take a deep breath in and at the same time angle the probe cranially under the costal margin to scan through the liver.
- Take note of the liver characteristics listed in Step 4.
- Look specifically for the hepatic veins and their confluence at the IVC.
- Take representative images of the right, middle and left hepatic veins.

11. TS: liver – level of porta hepatis

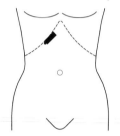

- Keep the probe parallel to the right costal margin.
- Ask the patient to take a deep breath in again. At the same time, angle the probe cranially under the costal margin, and sweep cranially then caudally to scan through the liver in TS.
- Take note of the liver characteristics listed in Step 4.
- Specifically examine the porta hepatis area for lymph nodes.
- Take representative image(s).

12. TS: liver – level of right kidney

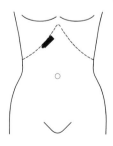

- Keep the probe parallel to the right costal margin.
- Ask the patient to take a deep breath in again. At the same time, angle the probe cranially under the costal margin, and sweep cranially then caudally to scan through the liver in TS.
- Take note of the liver characteristics listed in Step 4.
- Specifically examine the liver at the level of the right kidney.
- Make sure to scan inferiorly off the liver.
- Take representative image(s).

What to look for

Scan image

10.

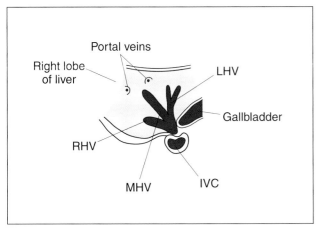

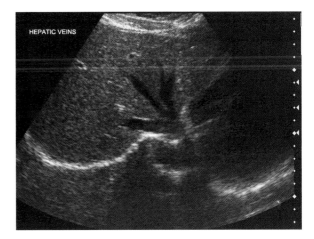

11.

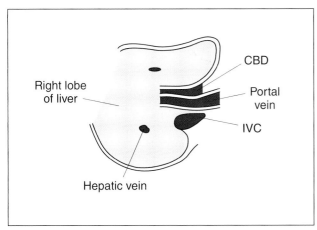

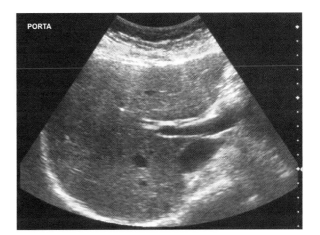

12.

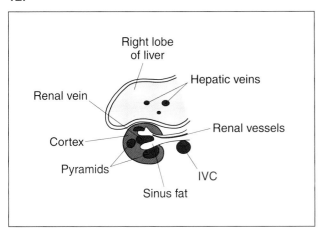

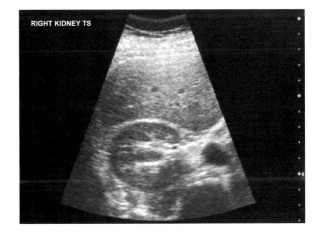

Probe position

13. LS: gallbladder

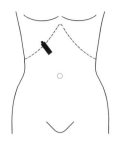

Instructions

- Scan in the RUQ to find the GB – position varies in different patients.
- Rotate the probe so that the GB is imaged in its long axis.
- Now keep the probe face over the same area of skin, but angle the probe handle backwards and forwards to scan through the whole GB.
- Narrow the sector width and use multiple focal zones with or without zoom to improve detail.
- Take note of:
  - GB contents: calculi, sludge, polyps, gas, mass?
  - GB wall thickness (<3 mm?)
  - pericholecystic fluid
  - localized tenderness (Murphy's sign)
- If something can be seen within the GB, try moving the patient and rescanning to see if it has moved with gravity (calculi/sludge vs polyp/mass).
- Measure any abnormalities seen.
- Acquire at least three representative images.

14. TS: gallbladder

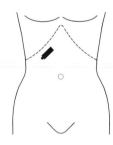

- Scan the GB in TS: to do this, first scan it in LS and then rotate the probe anticlockwise through 90° to image in TS.
- Now keep the probe face over the same area of skin, but angle the probe handle backwards and forwards to scan through the whole GB in TS.
- Narrow the sector width and use multiple focal zones with or without zoom to improve detail.
- Take note of the GB characteristics listed in Step 13.
- If something can be seen within the GB, try moving the patient and rescanning to see if it has moved with gravity (calculi/sludge vs polyp/mass).
- Measure any abnormalities seen.
- Acquire at least three representative images.

What to look for

Scan image

13.

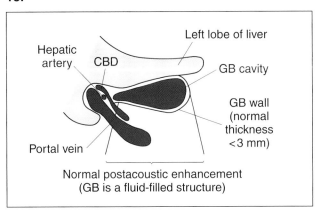

- Hepatic artery
- CBD
- Left lobe of liver
- GB cavity
- GB wall (normal thickness <3 mm)
- Portal vein
- Normal postacoustic enhancement (GB is a fluid-filled structure)

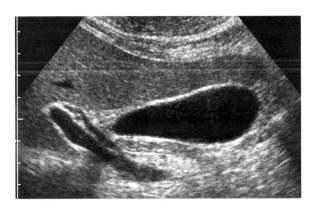

14.

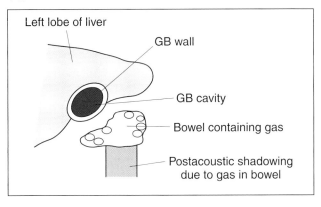

- Left lobe of liver
- GB wall
- GB cavity
- Bowel containing gas
- Postacoustic shadowing due to gas in bowel

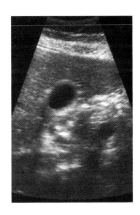

Probe position	*Instructions*

15. LS: right kidney

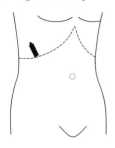

- Turn the patient 45° onto the left side.
- Place the probe in the RUQ and ask the patient to breathe in and hold.
- Locate the right kidney in LS. If there is difficulty finding it, try a more posterolateral approach. If rib shadows interfere, try scanning with the probe angled along a rib space.
- Scan through the kidney in LS, observing:
  - cortical thickness and echogenicity
  - medullary pyramids
  - pelvicalyceal system
- Are there any masses, cysts, calculi or hydronephrosis?
- Measure any abnormalities seen.
- Measure the greatest kidney length (pole-to-pole).
- Acquire at least two representative images.

16. TS: right kidney

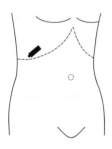

- Turn the probe 90° anticlockwise to scan in TS.
- Narrow the FOV and use two focal zones, with the second at the posterior aspect of the kidney.
- Ask the patient to breathe in and hold.
- Scan through the right kidney in TS and take note of the kidney characteristics listed in Step 15.
- If bowel gas shadows interfere, ask the patient to push out abdomen or press over the kidney with your free hand to displace the bowel.
- Measure any abnormalities seen.
- Acquire at least two representative images.

17. LS: spleen

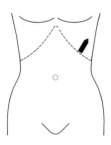

- Ask the patient to lie either 45° onto the right side or supine. It is best to scan the spleen with the patient gently breathing. To find the spleen, place the probe in the 9th ICS AAL.
- Sweep the probe posteriorly and anteriorly to scan through the whole spleen in LS.
- Take note of:
  - echogenicity compared with the left kidney (the spleen should be brighter)
  - texture (fine homogenous = normal)
  - any masses/infarcts/varices
- Measure the spleen size from tip to tip.
- Acquire representative image(s).

What to look for

15.

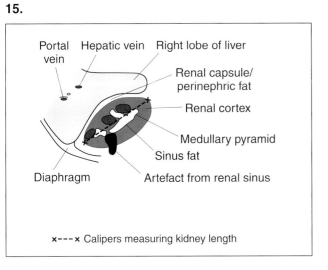

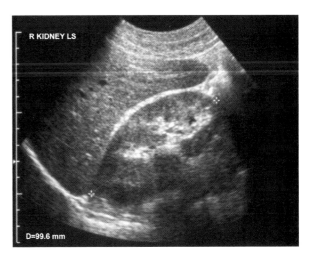

16.

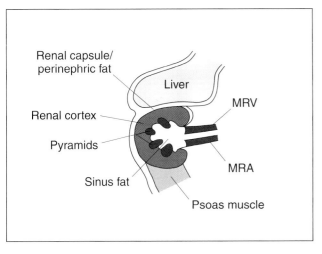

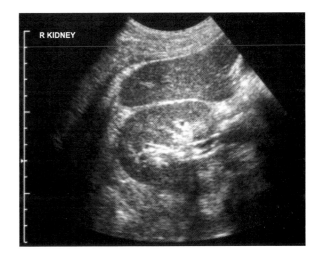

17.

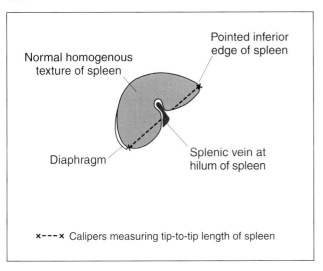

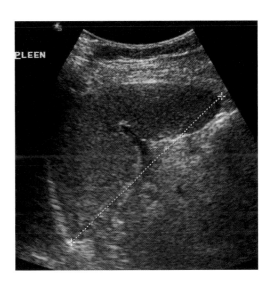

Probe position	**Instructions**

18. TS: spleen

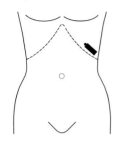

- Find the spleen in LS and then rotate the probe through 90° anticlockwise to image it in TS.
- Sweep the probe superiorly and inferiorly to scan through the whole spleen.
- Take note of the spleen characteristics listed in Step 17.
- Measure any abnormalities seen.
- Acquire representative image(s).

19. LS: left kidney

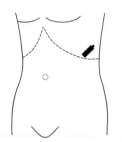

- Turn the patient 45° onto the right side.
- Place the probe obliquely over the LUQ and ask the patient to breathe in and hold.
- Look for the left kidney in LS with the spleen adjacent to it for comparison of echogenicity (the spleen should be brighter).
  Hint: the left kidney is higher and more posterior than the right – the 11th ICS is a good landmark.
- Scan through the left kidney in LS, observing:
  - cortical thickness and echogenicity
  - medullary pyramids
  - pelvicalyceal system
- Are there any masses, cysts, calculi or hydronephrosis?
- Measure any abnormalities seen.
- Measure the greatest kidney length (pole-to-pole).
- Acquire at least two representative images.

20. TS: left kidney

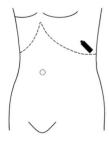

- Turn the probe 90° anticlockwise to scan in TS.
- Narrow the FOV and use two focal zones with the second at the posterior aspect of kidney.
- Ask the patient to breathe in and hold.
- Scan through the left kidney in TS and take note of the kidney characteristics listed in Step 19.
- If bowel gas shadows interfere, ask the patient to push their abdomen out or press over the kidney with your free hand to displace the bowel.
- Measure any abnormalities seen.
- Acquire at least two representative images.

What to look for

Scan image

18.

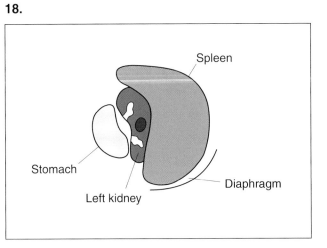

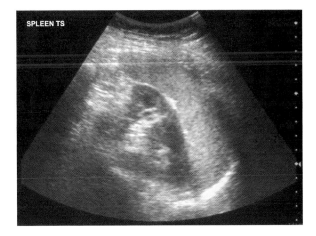

19.

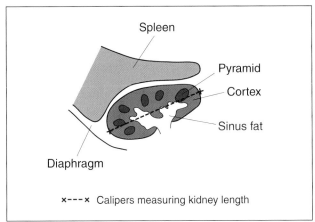

x---x Calipers measuring kidney length

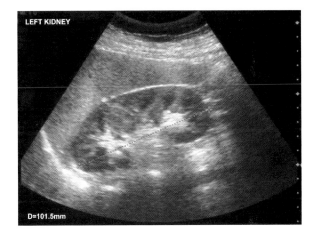

20.

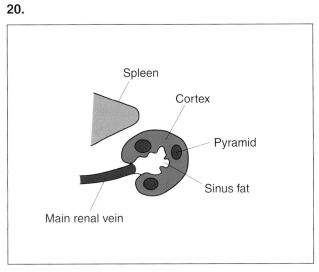

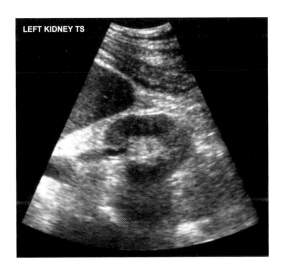

ABDOMEN PROTOCOL A

Below is a summary of the abdomen protocol described in this chapter. Protocol A is just one of many different protocols that can be used. On the following pages, other suggested abdomen protocols are summarized, with a list of advantages and disadvantages for each one. They differ in the *sequence* of images but they all encompass a whole examination of the abdomen in at least two planes. We recommend that an operator should pick one of the protocols, learn it and stick to it – that way nothing will be missed out. The bottom line is that it does not really matter which protocol is used, as long as you are methodical, consistent and thorough.

Midline	1. TS: pancreas
	2. LS: pancreas
	3. TS: aorta
	4. TS: left lobe of liver
LS: sweep across RUQ	5. LS: aorta and left lobe of the liver
	6. LS: IVC and caudate
	7. LS: porta hepatis and CBD
	8. LS: right liver medial to right kidney
	9. LS: right kidney/liver
TS: liver	10. Level of hepatic veins
	11. Level of porta hepatis
	12. Level of right kidney
Gallbladder	13. LS
	14. TS
Right kidney	15. LS
	16. TS
Spleen	17. LS
	18. TS
Left kidney	19. LS
	20. TS

ABDOMEN PROTOCOL B

LS sweep across RUQ
    1. Liver/right kidney
    2. Liver medial to right kidney
    3. Porta hepatis
    4. CBD (and measurement)
    5. IVC and caudate
    6. Aorta and left lobe of liver

Midline
    7. LS: left lobe of liver
    8. LS: pancreas
    9. LS: aorta
    10. TS: pancreas
    11. TS: aorta

TS liver
    12. Left lobe of liver
    13. Level of hepatic veins/IVC
    14. Level of porta hepatis
    15. Level of right kidney

Gallbladder
    16. LS
    17. TS

Right kidney
    18. LS
    19. TS

Spleen
    20. LS
    21. TS

Left kidney
    22. LS
    23. TS

ABDOMEN PROTOCOL C

Pancreas	1. TS
	2. LS
Liver LS	3. LS: left lobe of liver
	4. LS: IVC and caudate
	5. LS: porta hepatis and CBD
	6. LS: right lobe of liver
Right kidney	7. LS
	8. TS
Liver TS	9. Right lobe at level of hepatic veins
	10. Right lobe at level of porta hepatis
	11. Left lobe of liver
Gallbladder	12. LS
	13. TS
Spleen	14. LS
	15. TS
Left kidney	16. LS
	17. TS
Aorta	18. TS

EVALUATION OF ABDOMEN PROTOCOLS

Protocol	Advantages	Disadvantages
A	• There is an improved chance of visualizing the midline structures • Visualizing the pancreas is a confidence booster • Small amounts of ascites will have had time to accumulate in the hepatorenal space	• It is not possible to set up the system to assess liver echotexture – especially in patients with a 'fatty liver', when the left lobe may be echo-bright. In this case, the overall gain may be reduced to assess this lobe. Then, when the right lobe is assessed, the overall gain must be increased. As a result, it may not be possible to determine which lobe is abnormal
B	• It allows an initial comparison of echogenicity of liver/right kidney. Any variation from this throughout the liver may then be noted • The size of the liver is known immediately • A plan of the scan – all-intercostal for right lobe or a combination of sub-/intercostal – can be made • An immediate note of moderate/large amount of ascites can be made	• Repeat inspiration and breathhold techniques may lead to midline structures being obscured by bowel gas • Small amounts of ascites may not have accumulated in the dependent hepatorenal space
C	• There is an improved chance of visualizing the pancreas (a confidence booster) • Viewing all right-sided structures in LS first and then in TS is simple to remember • Fewer probe rotations are needed, which can speed up scan time • Small amounts of ascites will have had time to accumulate in the hepatorenal space	• It is less sensitive for subtle abnormalities of liver echotexture • Liver scanning is interrupted to look at right kidney. With this discontinuity, it is important to review any suspicious areas seen in the LS liver images

LIVER: PATHOLOGY

1. Hepatomegaly

Common causes are malignancy, infection and right heart failure.

Ultrasound features

- Segment 6 of the liver extends below the inferior pole of the right kidney (in LS)
- Segment 6 has a rounded margin (i.e. angle >45°)
- Both right and left lobes tend to be enlarged

Hint: Do not confuse hepatomegaly with Riedel's lobe (a congenitally large segment 6).

Ultrasound features of Riedel's lobe

- Segment 6 of the liver extends beyond the inferior pole of the right kidney (in LS)
- Segment 6 has a pointed margin (i.e. angle <45°)
- The left lobe of the liver tends to be small

2. Fatty liver (hepatic steatosis)

Fatty infiltration of the liver is a very common finding. Causes include obesity, alcoholism and diabetes. It can be diffuse or focal. If focal, it is usually found in segment 4, adjacent to the porta.

Ultrasound features
- Bigger liver
- Brighter liver (i.e. much brighter than renal cortex)
- Loss of portal vein wall definition
- Postattenuation fallout

What to look for	*Scan image*

1a. Hepatomegaly

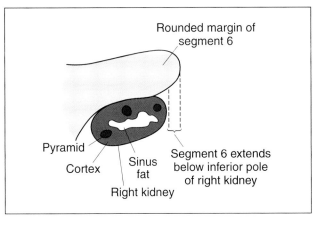

Rounded margin of segment 6

Segment 6 extends below inferior pole of right kidney

Pyramid

Cortex

Sinus fat

Right kidney

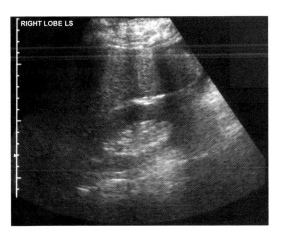

RIGHT LOBE LS

1b. Riedel's lobe

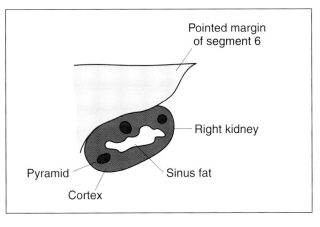

Pointed margin of segment 6

Right kidney

Pyramid

Sinus fat

Cortex

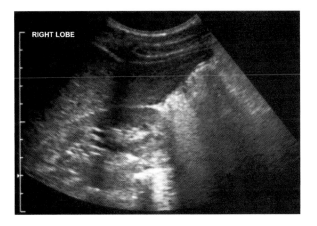

RIGHT LOBE

2. Fatty liver

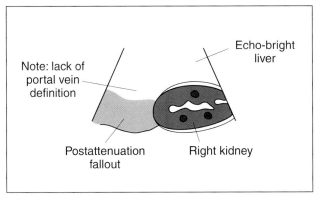

Echo-bright liver

Note: lack of portal vein definition

Postattenuation fallout

Right kidney

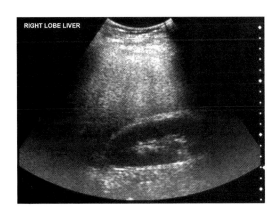

RIGHT LOBE LIVER

3. Focal fat sparing

Just as a normal liver can have focal fatty infiltration, sometimes a diffusely fat liver can have focal sparing.

Ultrasound features

- Usually affects segments 1 or 4
- Is seen as a relatively echo-poor area
- Has an irregular edge
- Has no mass effect
- May mimic a cyst

4. Metastases

Liver metastases are commonly from a primary malignancy of colon, stomach, breast or lung.

Ultrasound features

- Wide variation in appearance
- May be single or multiple, cystic or solid
- Echo-poor, echo-bright or a mass of mixed echogenicity
- Gastrointestinal primary tumours commonly give echo-bright metastases. These can have a 'target' appearance due to an echo-poor rim of oedema
- Exhibit mass effect with disruption of normal anatomy
- Occasionally show neovascularization (tortuous new vessels seen with colour Doppler)

What to look for

3. Focal fatty sparing

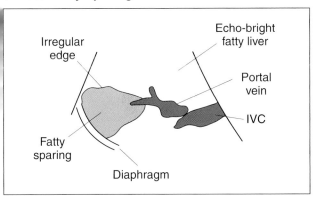

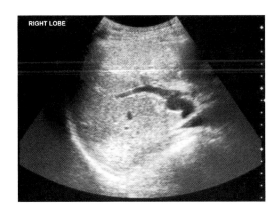

4a. Liver metastases

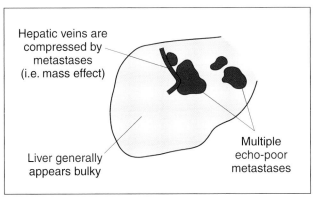

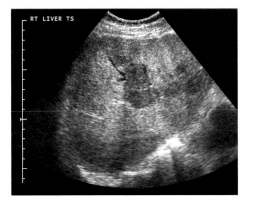

4b. Liver metastases

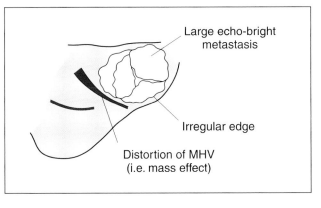

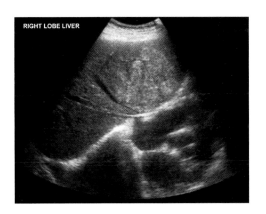

5. Cirrhosis

This is chronic liver disease resulting in fibrosis of liver parenchyma and nodule formation. Alcohol is the most common cause followed by chronic hepatitis B and C infection.

Ultrasound features

- Small contracted liver
- Irregular and nodular surface
- Increased parenchymal echotexture, which can be:
  - coarse, i.e. micronodular cirrhosis
  - contain discrete echo-poor nodules >1 cm: i.e. macronodular cirrhosis
- Also look carefully for:
  - evidence of portal hypertension: ascites; splenomegaly; varices
  - associated hepatocellular carcinoma

What to look for	*Scan image*

5a. Early cirrhosis

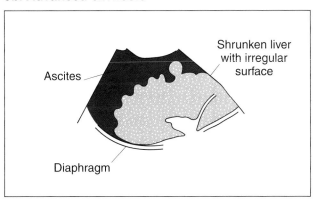

Skin and fat

Small amount of ascites

Coarse echotexture of liver

Diaphragm

Right kidney

Perinephric fat

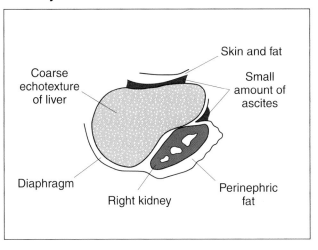

5b. Advanced cirrhosis

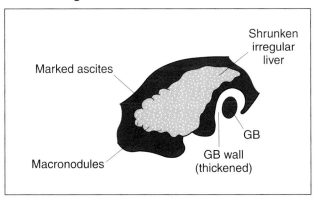

Ascites

Shrunken liver with irregular surface

Diaphragm

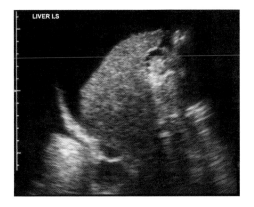

5c. End-stage cirrhosis

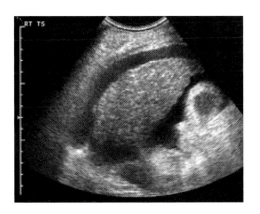

Marked ascites

Shrunken irregular liver

Macronodules

GB

GB wall (thickened)

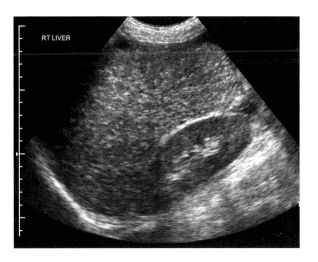

6. Hepatocellular carcinoma

This is the most common primary liver cancer. The majority of HCCs occur in cirrhotic livers (see Page 40) which can make their detection very difficult due to the background changes.

Ultrasound features

- Usually in a cirrhotic liver
- Small HCCs are echo-poor
- Larger HCCs are echo-bright due to internal haemorrhage and necrosis
- Diffuse HCCs cause a generalized echotexture abnormality and can be easily missed
- Look for indirect evidence of tumour e.g. localised surface bulge

Hint: Always look for tumour thrombus within the portal and hepatic veins, and check for the patency of flow within these vessels (60% invade the PV; 25% invade HVs).

7. Hepatic cysts

These can be congenital or acquired. They are of no clinical significance unless associated with PCKD.

Ultrasound features

- Smooth edge
- Thin wall
- Echo-free contents
- Postacoustic enhancement

What to look for	**Scan image**

6a. Single HCC

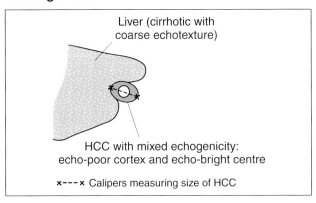

Liver (cirrhotic with coarse echotexture)

HCC with mixed echogenicity: echo-poor cortex and echo-bright centre

x---x Calipers measuring size of HCC

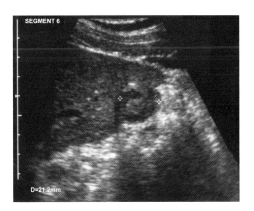

6b. Multiple HCCs

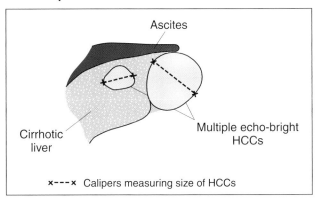

Ascites

Cirrhotic liver

Multiple echo-bright HCCs

x---x Calipers measuring size of HCCs

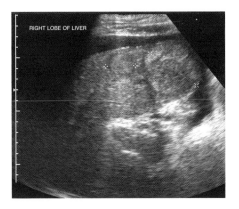

7. Simple hepatic cyst

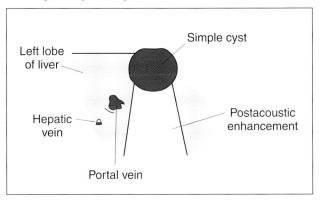

Left lobe of liver

Simple cyst

Hepatic vein

Postacoustic enhancement

Portal vein

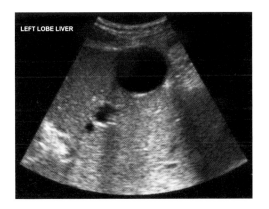

8. Liver abscess

This is a localized collection of pus within the liver. The majority are pyogenic and secondary to ascending infection, e.g. cholangitis, diverticulitis etc. They can also result from bloodborne sepsis such as endocarditis. Rarely are they caused by amoebic or hydatid disease.

Ultrasound features

- Irregular wall
- Echo-poor lesion
- Contain 'lumpy' echo-bright debris
- Display variable postacoustic enhancement
- If the abscess contains gas intense reverberations are seen.

9. Haemangioma

These are benign vascular lesions comprising multiple tiny blood vessels. They are a common incidental finding (5% of population). 80% occur in females.

Ultrasound features

- Usually small (<4 cm) well-defined echo-bright lesions
- Can appear echo-poor
- Postacoustic enhancement is common
- Slowly flowing blood – therefore appear avascular with colour/power Doppler

10. Congestive cardiac failure (or right heart failure alone)

The commonest causes are ischaemic heart disease, hypertension and COPD.

Ultrasound features

- Dilated hepatic veins
- Dilated IVC (>2 cm AP diameter)
- Loss of IVC movement with respiration

What to look for   *Scan image*

8. Liver abscess (and drain in situ)

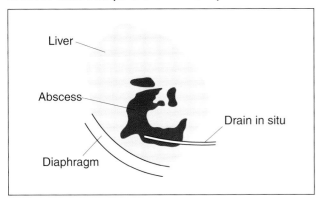

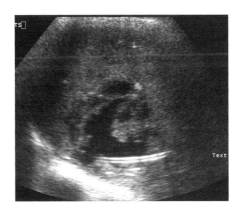

9. Haemangioma

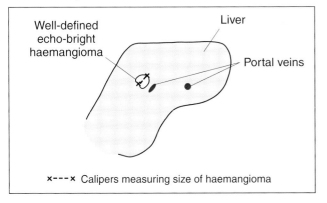

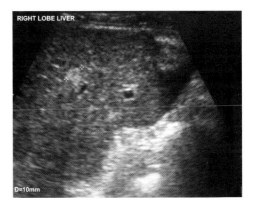

10. Congestive cardiac failure

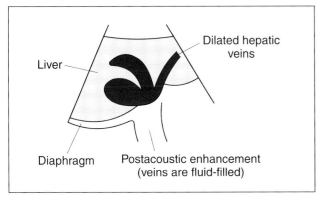

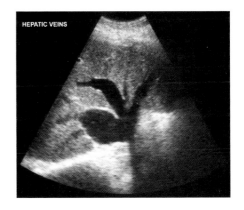

GALLBLADDER AND BILIARY TREE: PATHOLOGY

1. Gallstones

Cholesterol stones

- Risk factors: 'female, fat, over forty'
- Characteristics: large solitary stone

Pigmented stones

- Risk factors: haemolysis (consider in patients with sickle cell disease)
- Characteristics: small, irregular and multiple

Ultrasound features

- Echo-bright
- Well-defined
- Postacoustic shadowing
- Move to most dependent part with change in patient's position (cf. polyps)

2. Cholecystitis

This is infection of the gallbladder. 95% of cases have gallstones; 5% have sludge; acalculous cholecystitis (in ICU patients) is rare.

Ultrasound features

- Tender gallbladder
- Murphy's sign positive – patient catches breath on deep inspiration as gallbladder descends pushing against the probe
- Presence of stones or sludge (>95% of cases)
- Gallbladder wall thickness >3 mm
- Oedematous wall with indistinct outline
- Rim of echo-free pericholecystic fluid (also look in Morrison's pouch for free fluid)

What to look for

1a. Gallstone

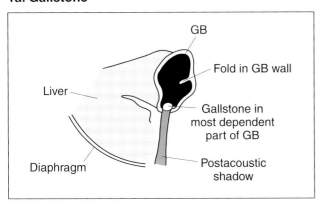

1b. Biliary sludge

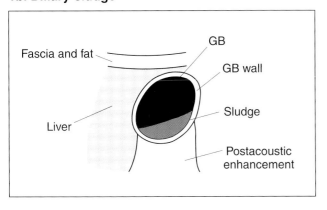

2. Cholecystitis

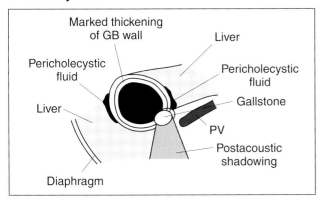

Scan image

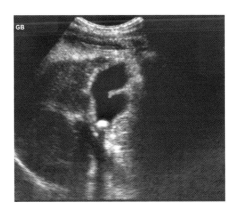

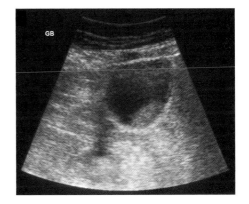

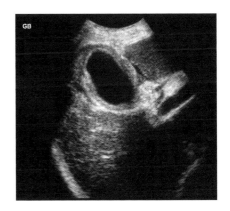

3. Biliary obstruction

Most common causes

- Intrinsic: gallstones, cholangiocarcinoma, stricture, sclerosing cholangitis
- Extrinsic: acute pancreatitis, lymph nodes, carcinoma of the head of the pancreas

Ultrasound features

- 'Double-barelled shotgun' sign of dilated bile duct radicals parallel to PV branches in the liver
- Dilation of ducts proximal to the obstruction
- If obstruction is distal the CBD will also be dilated (>6 mm or >9 mm postcholecystectomy)
- Ampullary obstruction (e.g. pancreatic carcinoma) causes 'double duct' sign of dilated CBD and dilated pancreatic duct (>2 mm)
- Look carefully for cause of obstruction e.g. gallstones, tumour

4. Gallbladder polyps

These occur in 5% of the population, and are usually asymptomatic. They are usually benign, but need monitoring as there is a risk of carcinoma developing in larger polyps.

Ultrasound features

- Echo-bright and well-defined
- No postacoustic shadowing
- Sometimes on a stalk
- Do not move to the most dependent part of the gallbladder (cf. gallstones)

Hint: Sit the patient up and rescan to see if the polyp/stone etc. has moved.

What to look for	*Scan image*

3a. Biliary obstruction: stone in CBD

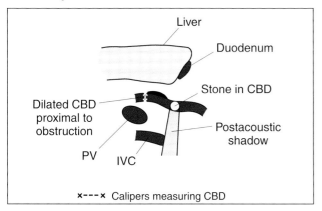

Liver
Duodenum
Stone in CBD
Dilated CBD proximal to obstruction
Postacoustic shadow
PV
IVC
×---× Calipers measuring CBD

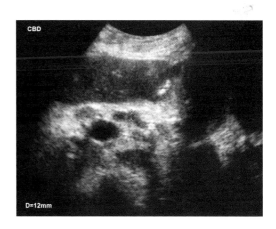

3b. Biliary obstruction: dilated CBD

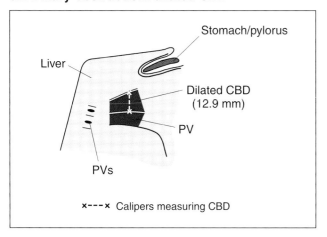

Stomach/pylorus
Liver
Dilated CBD (12.9 mm)
PV
PVs
×---× Calipers measuring CBD

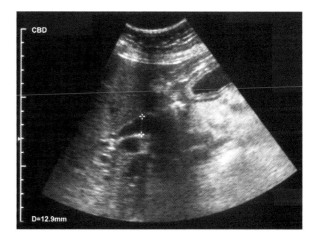

4. Gallbladder polyps

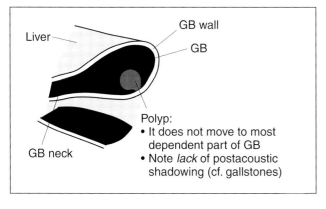

Liver
GB wall
GB
Polyp:
• It does not move to most dependent part of GB
• Note *lack* of postacoustic shadowing (cf. gallstones)
GB neck

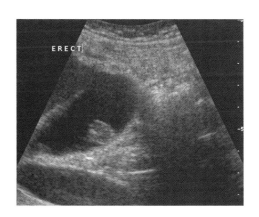

5. Adenomyomatosis

This benign condition is associated with gallstones. There is hyperplasia of the gallbladder wall epithelium resulting in mucosal diverticulae that extend into the muscular layer. The diverticulae are seen within the wall as fluid- or crystal-filled spaces.

Ultrasound features

- GB wall thickening can be diffuse or focal
- Diverticulae containing bile are echo-poor
- Diverticulae containing stones/sludge give a 'comet tail' artefact

6. Cholecystic carcinoma

This uncommon gastrointestinal malignancy has an increased prevalence in women and the elderly.

Ultrasound features

- Often associated with gallstones
- Gallbladder wall thickening in early disease
- GB is replaced by a mass of mixed echogenicity in later disease

7. Pneumobilia

This is air in the biliary tree. The commonest causes are iatrogenic (surgery, ERCP, etc.), cholecystenteric fistula and gallstone ileus.

Ultrasound features

- Reflective linear echoes within the biliary tree
- Ill-defined reverberation shadows seen posterior to the air

What to look for

5. Adenomyomatosis

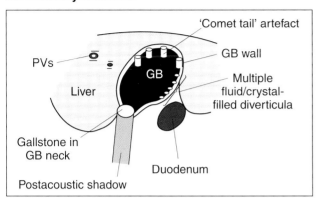

'Comet tail' artefact
GB wall
Multiple fluid/crystal-filled diverticula
PVs
GB
Liver
Duodenum
Gallstone in GB neck
Postacoustic shadow

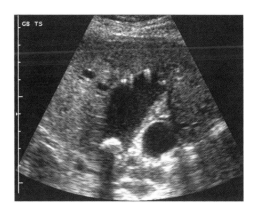

6. Cholecystic carcinoma

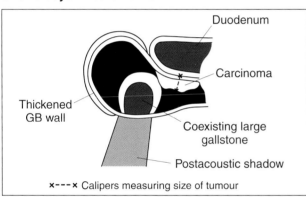

Duodenum
Carcinoma
Thickened GB wall
Coexisting large gallstone
Postacoustic shadow
x---x Calipers measuring size of tumour

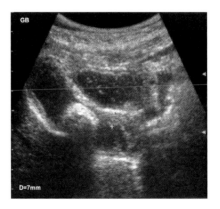

7. Pneumobilia

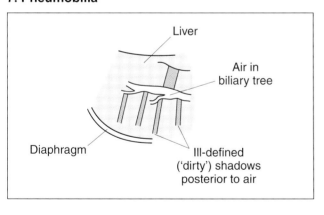

Liver
Air in biliary tree
Diaphragm
Ill-defined ('dirty') shadows posterior to air

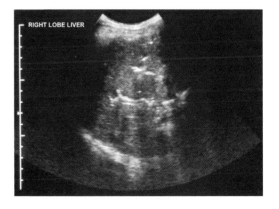

PANCREAS: PATHOLOGY

1. Acute pancreatitis

The most common causes are alcohol, gallstones, steroids, autoimmune causes and trauma.

Ultrasound features

- Swollen/enlarged pancreas
- Echo-poor and difficult to visualize
- Tender over midline
- Fluid in flanks

2. Chronic pancreatitis

The most common cause is chronic alcohol abuse. Rarer causes include pancreatic duct obstruction (stone, carcinoma), cystic fibrosis, haemochromatosis and familial causes.

Ultrasound features

- Small atrophic echo-bright pancreas
- Speckled calcification
- Dilated pancreatic duct (60% cases)

Three causes of an echo-bright pancreas
- Advanced age
- Cystic fibrosis
- Chronic pancreatitis

3. Pancreatic carcinoma

This occurs usually in patients >40 years old. It presents with pain radiating through to the back, with or without jaundice. 65% of carcinomas are found in the head of the pancreas (>body>tail).

Ultrasound features

- Irregular mass
- Usually echo-poor
- Disruption of normal anatomy
- Double-duct sign (i.e. dilated CBD and pancreatic duct)

What to look for

1. Acute pancreatitis

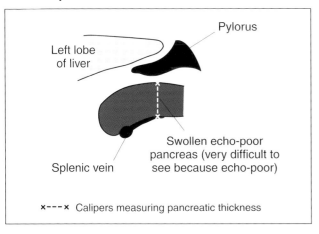

Left lobe of liver

Pylorus

Splenic vein

Swollen echo-poor pancreas (very difficult to see because echo-poor)

×---× Calipers measuring pancreatic thickness

2. Chronic pancreatitis

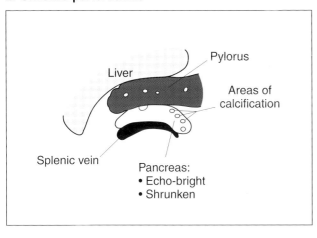

Liver

Pylorus

Areas of calcification

Splenic vein

Pancreas:
• Echo-bright
• Shrunken

3. Pancreatic carcinoma

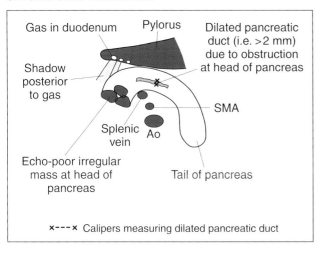

Gas in duodenum

Pylorus

Dilated pancreatic duct (i.e. >2 mm) due to obstruction at head of pancreas

Shadow posterior to gas

SMA

Splenic vein

Ao

Echo-poor irregular mass at head of pancreas

Tail of pancreas

×---× Calipers measuring dilated pancreatic duct

Scan image

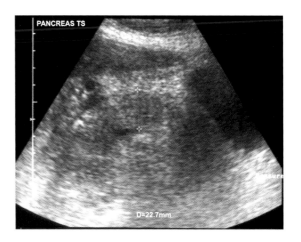

PANCREAS TS

D=22.7mm

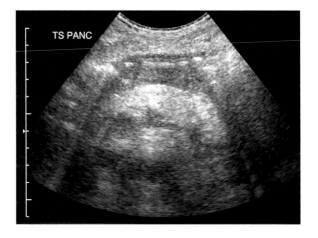

TS PANC

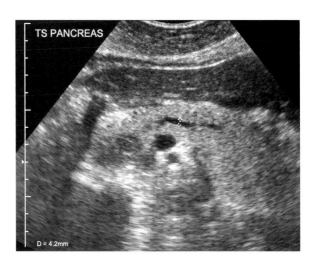

TS PANCREAS

D = 4.2mm

SPLEEN: PATHOLOGY

1. Splenunculus

This is accessory spleen tissue. It occurs in 10% of the population, and is an incidental finding of no clinical significance.

Ultrasound features

- Spherical
- Well-defined smooth outline
- Same echogenicity and echotexture as spleen
- Usually found at hilum

2. Splenomegaly

The most common causes in the UK are portal hypertension, malignancy (lymphoma, leukaemia, myelofibrosis) and infection.

Ultrasound features

- >13 cm when measured from inferior pole tip to superior pole tip
- Inferior margin becomes rounded
- Look for clues as to the cause e.g. ascites, cirrhosis, lymph nodes

3. Lymphoma

This is the most common malignancy of the spleen.

Ultrasound features

- Splenomegaly
- Associated lymphadenopathy in abdomen
- Solitary or multiple echo-poor lesions in the splenic parenchyma

| **What to look for** | **Scan image** |

1. Splenunculus

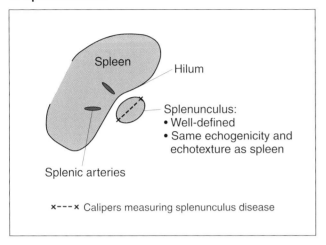

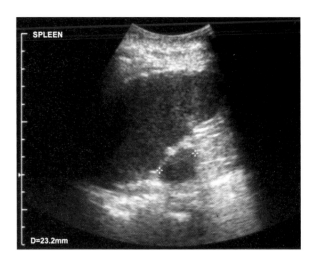

2. Splenomegaly

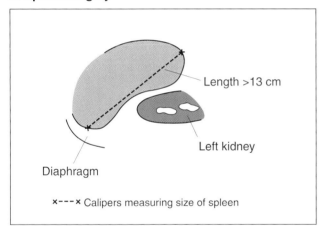

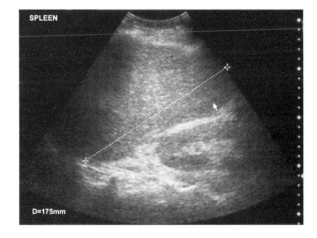

3. Lymphoma

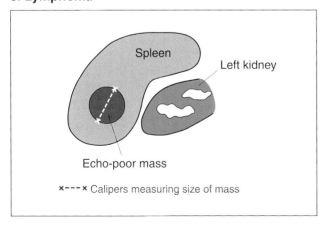

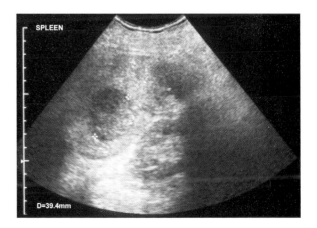

4

Renal, including renal transplant

ANATOMY

(i) LS anatomy and blood supply

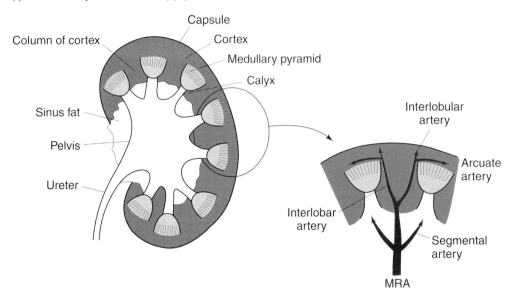

(ii) TS anatomy

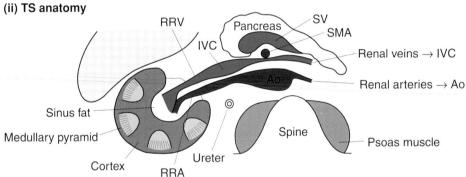

Key points

1. The kidneys lie obliquely, with the left about 2 cm higher than the right.
2. The normal LS length is 9–12 cm (lengths should not differ by >2 cm).
3. The normal cortical thickness is 1.5–2.5 cm (it thins with age).
4. The cortical echogenicity is normally slightly lower than that of the adjacent liver and spleen – mnemonic PLiSK!
5. The renal arteries arise from the aorta just inferior to the superior mesenteric artery at L2 level.

(iii) Transplant anatomy

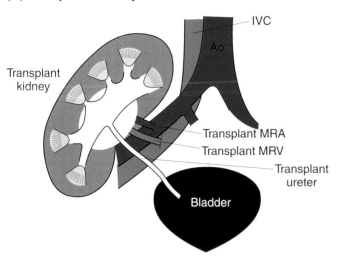

Key points

1. The kidney is transplanted into either iliac fossa (more often the right).
2. There are three anastomotic sites:
   - transplant MRA → iliac artery
   - transplant MRV → iliac vein
   - transplant ureter → bladder

PERFORMING THE SCAN

Step 1: Kidneys

- **Patient position**: Supine then turn 45° to each side.
- **Preparation**: Full bladder.
- **Probe**: Low-frequency (3–5 MHz) curvilinear.
- **Machine**: Select renal preset mode. Use two focal zones for TS imaging. Use tissue harmonics if the SNR is poor or with obese patients.
- **Method**: Acquire more than just representative images for each step if pathology is found.

Probe position

1. LS: right kidney/liver

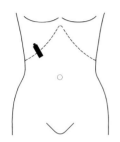

2. LS: right kidney

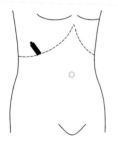

3. TS: right kidney

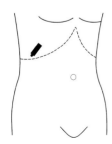

Instructions

- Begin by placing the probe obliquely in the RUQ.
- Ask the patient to breathe in and hold.
- Look for the right kidney in LS and adjacent liver (if there is difficulty, try a more posterolateral approach and/or turn the patient 45° to the left).
- Compare the echogenicity of the liver parenchyma and renal cortex (the liver should be a little brighter than the kidney – mnemonic PLiSK!).
- Look for any fluid in the hepatorenal space.
- Acquire a representative image.

- Now turn the patient 45° onto the left side.
- Ask the patient to breathe in and hold.
- Locate the right kidney in LS again.
- Scan through the kidney in LS, observing:
  - cortical thickness and echogenicity
  - medullary pyramids
  - pelvicalyceal system
- Are there any masses, cysts, calculi or hydronephrosis?
- If rib shadows interfere, try scanning with the probe angled along a rib space.
- Measure the greatest kidney length (pole-to-pole).
- Measure any abnormalities seen.
- Acquire a representative image.

- Turn the probe 90° anticlockwise to scan in TS.
- Narrow the FOV and use two focal zones, with the second at the posterior aspect of the kidney.
- Ask the patient to breathe in and hold.
- Scan through the right kidney in TS, observing for any pathology.
- If bowel gas shadows interfere, ask the patient to push out stomach or press over the kidney with your free hand to displace the bowel.
- Measure any abnormalities seen.
- Acquire a representative image.

What to look for

1.

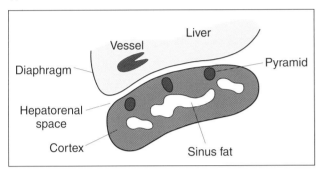

2.

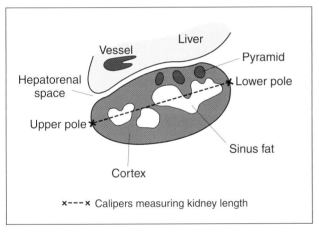

x---x Calipers measuring kidney length

3.

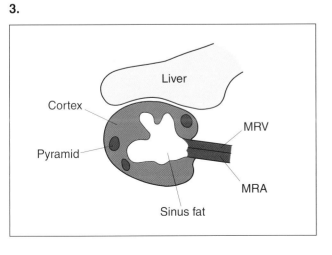

Scan image

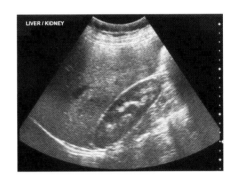

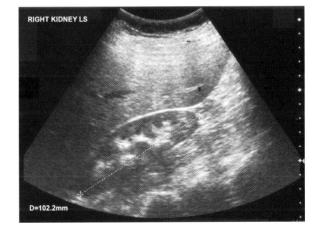

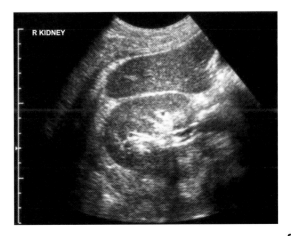

Probe position	**Instructions**

4. LS: left kidney/spleen

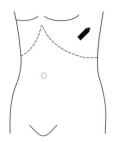

- Now turn the patient 45° onto the right side.
- Place the probe obliquely over the LUQ.
- Ask the patient to breathe in and hold.
- Look for the left kidney in LS with the spleen adjacent to it for comparison. (*Hint:* the left kidney is higher and more posterior than the right; the 11th intercostal space is a good landmark.)
- Compare the echogenicity of the spleen and the renal cortex (the spleen should be a little brighter than the kidney – mnemonic PLiSK!).
- Acquire a representative image.

5. LS: left kidney

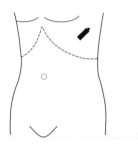

- Keep the probe in the same position.
- Scan through the left kidney in LS, observing:
  - cortical thickness and echogenicity
  - medullary pyramids
  - pelvicalyceal system
- Are there any masses, cysts, calculi or hydronephrosis?
- If rib shadows interfere, try scanning with the probe angled along a rib space.
- Measure the greatest kidney length (pole-to-pole).
- Acquire a representative image.

6. TS: left kidney

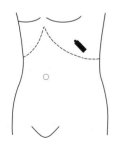

- Turn the probe 90° anticlockwise to scan in TS.
- Narrow the FOV and use two focal zones, with the second at the posterior aspect of the kidney.
- Ask the patient to breathe in and hold.
- Scan through the left kidney in TS, observing for any pathology.
- If bowel gas shadows interfere, ask the patient to push out the stomach or press over the kidney with your free hand to displace the bowel.
- Acquire a representative image.

If a kidney cannot be found, there are three possibilities:
1. It is present but hidden – e.g. a small atrophic kidney or an abundance of bowel gas.
2. It is in an ectopic location.
3. It is absent.

Each of these should be considered in conjunction with patient history, prior investigations, etc. in order to decide.

In patients over 50 years old, it is recommended to proceed to scan the aorta and measure its calibre, looking for an aortic aneurysm (see Chapter 5).

What to look for	*Scan image*

4.

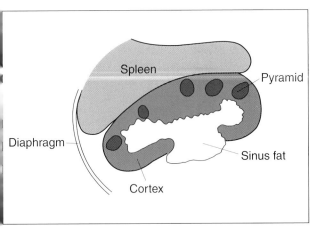

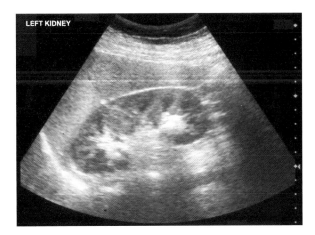

5.

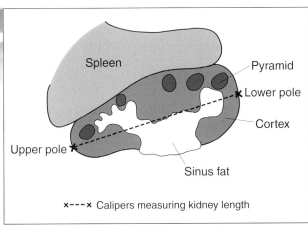

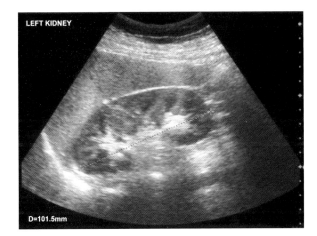

6.

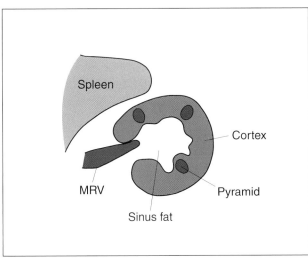

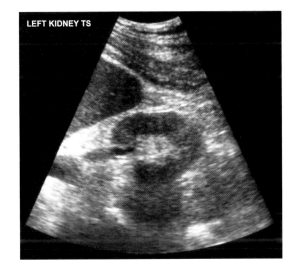

Step 2: Bladder

- **Patient position**: Supine.
- **Preparation**: Full bladder.
- **Probe**: Low-frequency (3–5 MHz) curvilinear.
- **Machine**: It is suggested that the tissue harmonics be turned on. Adjust the TGC to remove reverberation artefacts from the anterior bladder wall.
- **Method**: Acquire more than just representative images for each step if pathology is found.

Probe position	*Instructions*

7. LS: bladder

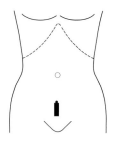

- Begin by placing the probe midline in the suprapubic area.
- Look for the bladder in LS and adjust the depth and FOV accordingly. (*Hint:* resting probe end on symphysis pubis often gives good views.)
- Scan across and through the bladder in LS, observing:
  - bladder wall thickness
  - bladder wall contour
  - any stones or debris?
- Acquire a representative image.

8. TS: bladder

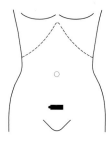

- Turn the probe 90° anticlockwise to scan in TS.
- Scan through the bladder in this plane, again looking for any pathology.
- Acquire a representative image.

9. Bladder volume

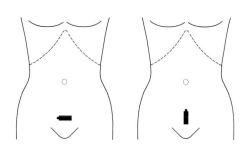

- Now calculate the bladder volume from the LS and TS images – the dual-image function (split screen) is helpful for this.
- Measure the LS craniocaudal diameter.
- Measure the TS transverse and AP diameters.
- Use the measurement package to calculate the volume (on most machines): volume = $A \times B \times C \times 0.53$.
- Acquire a representative image.

Ask the patient to void, and repeat these measurement steps to calculate the postmicturition volume.

TGC line adjustment

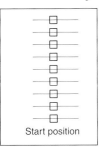

Start position

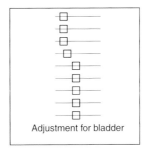

Adjustment for bladder

What to look for

Scan image

7.

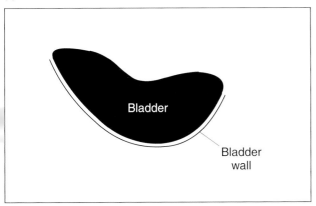

Bladder

Bladder wall

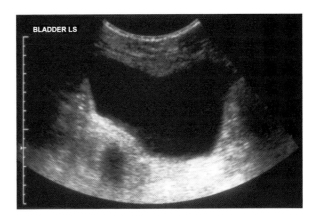

BLADDER LS

8.

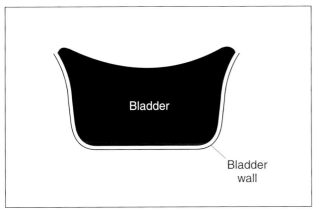

Bladder

Bladder wall

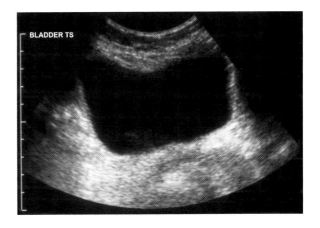

BLADDER TS

9.

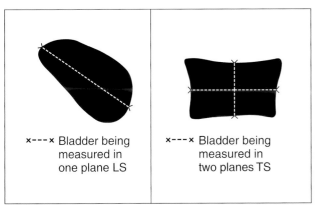

×- - -× Bladder being measured in one plane LS

×- - -× Bladder being measured in two planes TS

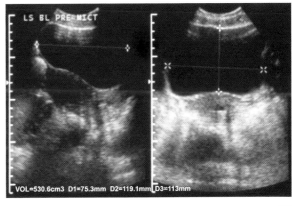

LS BL PRE-MICT

VOL=530.6cm3 D1=75.3mm D2=119.1mm D3=113mm

ASSESSING FOR RENAL ARTERY STENOSIS

Two methods can be used in ultrasound evaluation of RAS:

 (i) direct Doppler evaluation of the main renal arteries (MRAs)

(ii) indirect Doppler evaluation via interlobar artery waveforms

(i) Direct Doppler method

- **Patient position**: Turned 45° to right then left.
- **Preparation**: Fasted for 8 hours.
- **Probe**: Low-frequency (3–5 MHz) curvilinear.
- **Machine**: Select renal preset mode.

Probe position

1. LS measurements of both kidneys

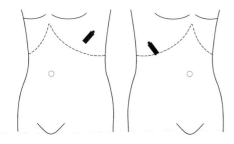

Instructions

- Begin with the patient turned 45° onto the right side. Place the probe obliquely over the LUQ. Ask the patient to breathe in and hold.
- Look for the left kidney in LS, adjusting as needed for rib/bowel gas interference.
- Measure its greatest length (pole-to-pole).
- Then turn the patient 45° onto the left side. Place the probe obliquely over the RUQ. Ask the patient to breathe in and hold.
- Look for the right kidney in LS.
- Measure its greatest length (pole-to-pole).
- Is there any significant (>2 cm) size difference?

2. Find the 'banana peel' window

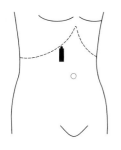

- Keeping the patient turned 45° to the left, place the probe in an LS position just right of the midline in the upper abdomen. Ask the patient to relax their abdominal wall muscles.
- Now slowly angle the probe towards the patient's left side, looking for the aorta and IVC in LS (use your free hand to displace obscuring bowel gas).
- With further probe manipulation, look for both renal arteries arising from the aorta at the 10 o'clock (right) and 4 o'clock (left) positions.
- This is the 'banana peel' window and is ideal for obtaining good MRA Doppler signals.

What to look for

1.

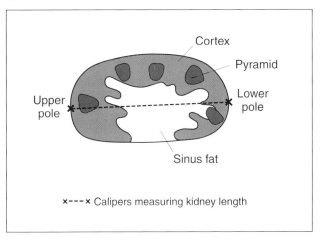

Scan image

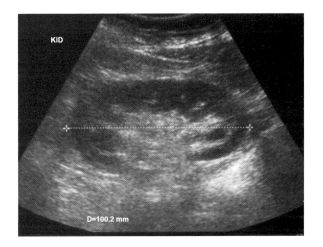

2.

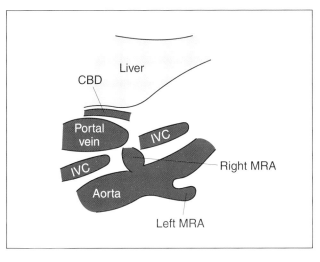

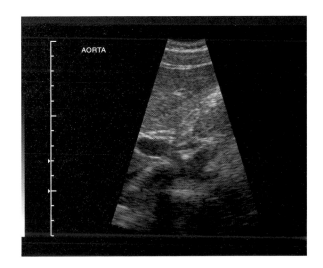

Probe position	*Instructions*

3. Spectral Doppler of MRAs and aorta

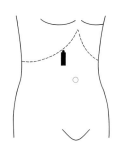

- Keeping this window in place, turn on colour Doppler and place the colour box over the aorta and MRAs.
- Optimize the colour signal: adjust the colour gain and focus position, narrow the FOV, reduce the colour box size, and set the filter at medium and the PRF at high.
- Identify the right MRA (flow towards probe).
- Turn on spectral Doppler and place the gate over this vessel, acquiring a trace. Optimize the waveform by adjusting the gate size and ensuring a beam-flow angle of 0°–60°.
- Measure the peak-systolic velocity.
- Identify the left MRA (flow away from probe).
- Acquire a spectral trace and peak velocity measurement of this vessel as above.
- Finally, acquire a trace of the aorta, as its peak velocity measurement is used to calculate the renal/aortic ratio (see below).

Criteria for diagnosing significant (>70%) RAS
- MRA peak-systolic velocity >180 cm/s
- Ratio of peak-systolic renal velocity to peak-systolic aortic velocity >3.5

(ii) Indirect Doppler method (via interlobar arteries)

- **Patient position**: Turned 45° to right then left.
- **Preparation**: Full bladder.
- **Probe**: Low-frequency (3–5 MHz) curvilinear.
- **Machine**: Select renal preset mode.

Probe position	*Instructions*

1. LS measurements of both kidneys

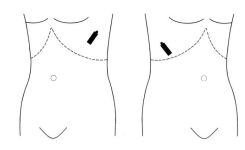

- Begin with the patient turned 45° onto the right side. Place the probe obliquely over the LUQ. Ask the patient to breathe in and hold.
- Look for the left kidney in LS, adjusting as needed for rib/bowel gas interference.
- Measure its greatest length (pole-to-pole).
- Then turn the patient 45° onto the left side. Place the probe obliquely over the RUQ. Ask the patient to breathe in and hold.
- Look for the right kidney in LS.
- Measure its greatest length (pole-to-pole).
- Is there any significant (>2 cm) size difference?

What to look for

3a. Colour Doppler over 'banana peel' window

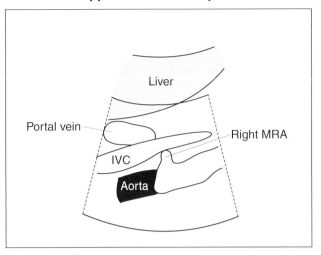

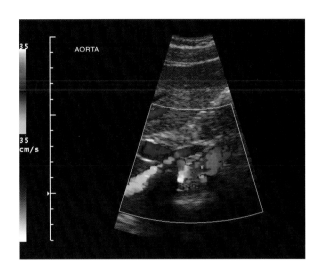

3b. Spectral Doppler of right MRA

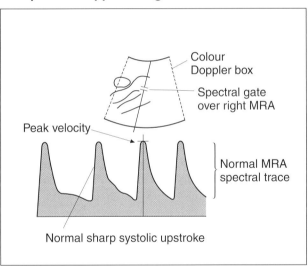

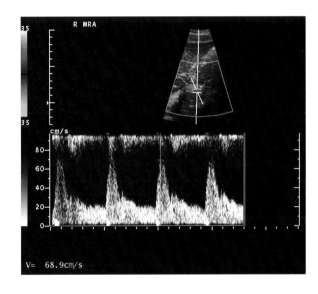

1.

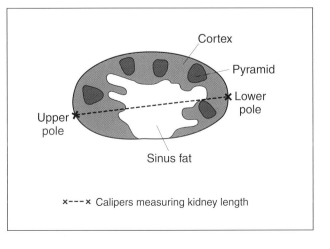

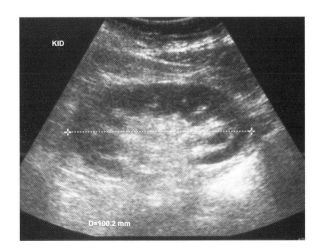

Probe position	*Instructions*
2. **LS interlobar artery spectral Doppler** 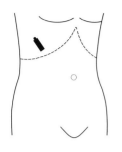	• Now move the probe slightly more posteriorly to visualize the right kidney in a more posterolateral LS section (see below). • Turn on colour Doppler and place the colour box over the upper pole region. • Optimize the colour signal: adjust the colour gain and focus position, narrow the FOV, reduce the colour box size, and set the PRF at high and the filter at medium. • Identify one of the interlobar arteries (running alongside the medullary pyramids). • Turn on spectral Doppler and place the gate over this vessel, acquiring a trace. Optimize the waveform by adjusting the gate size and ensuring a beam-flow angle of 0°–60° (the more posterolateral probe position helps with the angle-correct). • Select the calculation package (on most machines). Calculate the acceleration time via the interval from end-diastole to the *first* peak of the systolic upstroke. • Repeat this at the midzone and lower pole. • Then repeat for the left kidney.

Criteria for diagnosing significant (>70%) RAS
- Acceleration time (AT) >0.07 s
- AT >0.12 s gives a better positive predictive value
- Look for a 'parvus tardus' spectral wavefrom (see the pathology section for an example of this)

Both methods have their advantages and disadvantages, so a combination of the two is advised for optimal results:

Direct method

Advantages	*Disadvantages*
• A more sensitive test than indirect evaluation	• Technically very challenging, especially with obese patients • Difficult to detect an accessory renal artery, which may be the stenosed vessel and the cause of the patient's hypertension!

What to look for

2.

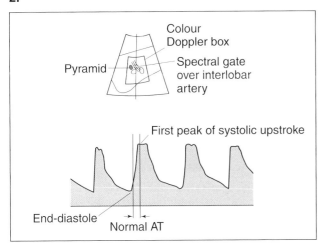

Scan image

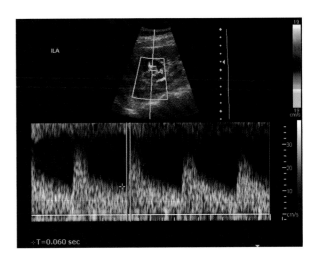

Indirect method

Advantages	Disadvantages
• Technically straightforward • If a stenosed accessory artery is present, it will often be detected by an abnormal waveform in the segment that it supplies	• Lack of sensitivity compared with the direct method • Coexistent intrinsic renal disease can make evaluation unreliable

RENAL TRANSPLANT SCAN

- **Patient position**: Supine.
- **Preparation**: Empty bladder.
- **Probe**: Low-frequency (3–5 MHz) curvilinear.
- **Machine**: Select renal preset mode. It is suggested that two focal zones are used.
- **Method**: Acquire more than just representative images for each step if pathology is found.

Probe position	*Instructions*

1. LS transplant

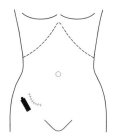

- Begin by placing the probe parallel and lateral to the iliac fossa scar (in RIF or LIF).
- Look for the transplant kidney in LS and adjust the depth and FOV accordingly.
- Scan through it in LS, then, turning the probe 90° anticlockwise, scan through it again in TS.
- Observe:
  - cortical echogenicity
  - corticomedullary differentiation
  - pelvicalyceal system dilation
  - any perirenal fluid collections?
- Acquire a representative image

Hint: If the system appears dilated, some centres advocate measuring the area of the kidney and the area of the renal pelvis, then using a dilation index program to grade severity.

2. LS interlobar artery spectral Doppler

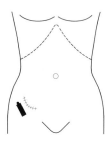

- Keep the probe in LS position.
- Turn on colour Doppler and place the colour box over the kidney.
- Optimize the colour signal: adjust the colour gain and focus position, narrow the FOV, reduce the colour box size, set the filter at low and adjust the PRF.
- Assess perfusion throughout the transplant – normally it should be to the cortical margins (power Doppler can also be used for this).
- Identify one of the interlobar arteries that run alongside the medullary pyramids.
- Turn on spectral Doppler and place the gate over this vessel, acquiring a trace. Optimize the waveform by adjusting the gate size and ensuring a beam-flow angle of 0°–60°.
- Select the calculation package (on most machines). Calculate the resistance index (RI) via the peak-systolic value S and the end-diastolic value D: $RI = (S - D)/S$.

Resistance index (RI)

- The normal transplant has a low-resistance arterial bed with RI <0.7
- Higher values imply intrinsic renal disease (e.g. rejection), but cannot specify disease type
- It is more helpful in transplants to record serial RI values for progression over time

---

What to look for

Scan image

1.

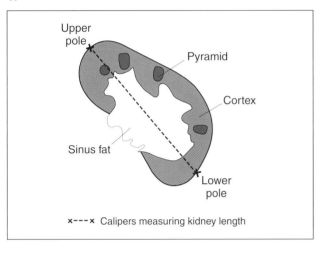

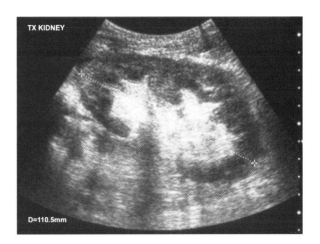

2a.

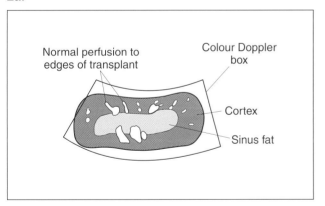

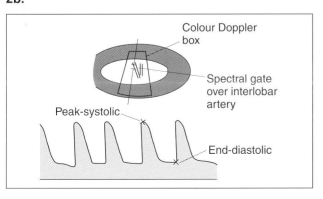

2b.

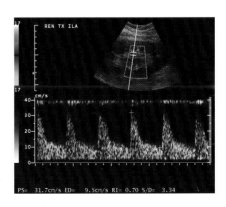

Probe position	**Instructions**

3. LS transplant MRA Doppler

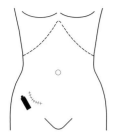

- Keep the probe in the LS position.
- Using colour Doppler, look for the MRA and MRV near the hilum, and if possible follow back to their anastomotic sites with the iliac vessels.
- Narrow the FOV; adjust the focus and colour box size to help with this.
- Identify the MRA (flow towards probe) coming off the iliac artery.
- Turn on spectral Doppler and place the gate over this vessel, acquiring a trace.
- Optimize the waveform by adjusting the gate size and ensuring a beam-flow angle of 0°–60°.
- Look for the normal sharp arterial systolic upstroke.
- Measure the peak-systolic flow velocity in this vessel (see below).
- Look for reverse (below baseline) end-diastolic flow on the trace – MRV thrombosis (see the pathology section for an example of this).

4. LS transplant MRV Doppler

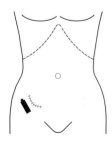

- Now identify the MRV (flow away from probe) coming off the iliac vein.
- Assess for patent flow in this vessel by acquiring a spectral Doppler trace from it.

Peak-systolic flow velocity in transplant MRA

- Velocities >250 cm/s are diagnostic for renal artery stenosis, which can occur at the anastomotic site
- This is a recognized cause of graft failure, and is usually treated with stenting

What to look for

Scan image

3a.

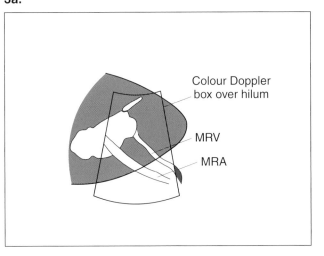

Colour Doppler box over hilum

MRV

MRA

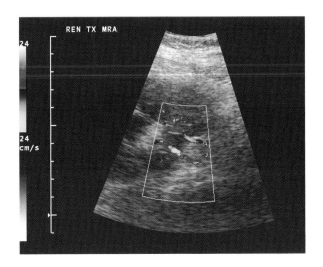

3b.

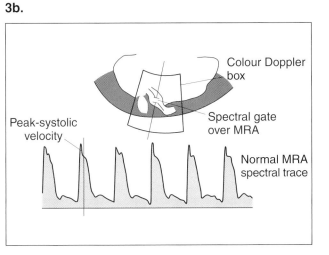

Colour Doppler box

Spectral gate over MRA

Peak-systolic velocity

Normal MRA spectral trace

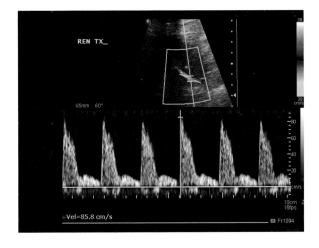

4.

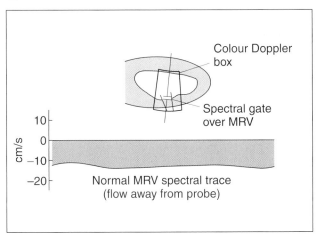

Colour Doppler box

Spectral gate over MRV

cm/s

Normal MRV spectral trace (flow away from probe)

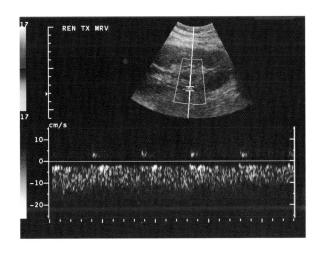

PATHOLOGY

1. Congenital variants

(a) Dromedary hump

This is a parenchymal prominence seen along the lateral border of the left kidney, usually just inferior to the spleen. It is important not to mistake this for a renal tumour.

(b) Column of Bertin

This is hypertrophy of a column of cortex that is seen protruding into the renal sinus fat. It is important to differentiate this from a renal tumour (the mass is in continuity with the cortex and is of the same echogenicity as the cortex).

(c) Horseshoe kidney

This is the most common renal fusion anomaly. The kidneys are connected across the midline at their lower poles by an isthmus of tissue. They are low-lying, as their normal ascent is restricted by the isthmus tethering on the inferior mesenteric artery. The lower poles are medially orientated and both renal pelvises lie anteriorly. Associated with an increased risk of stone formation, obstruction and infection, as well as certain renal tumours (e.g. Wilms' tumour).

(d) Duplex kidney

The collecting system is divided by a bridge of parenchymal tissue, with each half being drained by separate ureters. The ureter draining the upper-moiety inserts into the bladder inferior and medially to the lower-moiety ureter. It is associated with a ureterocele and is prone to obstruction. The lower-moiety ureter is prone to vesico-ureteric reflux, which can lead to chronic pyelonephritis. With ultrasound, the parenchymal bridge can be difficult to see. Hydronephrosis of one moiety (usually the upper) suggests the diagnosis.

What to look for

1a. Dromedary hump

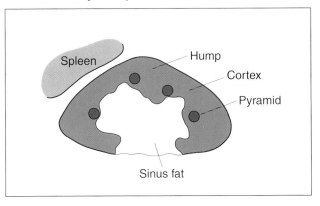

1b. Column of Bertin

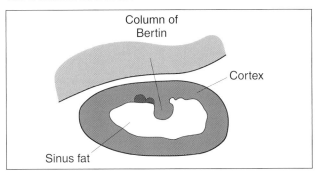

1c. Horseshoe kidney

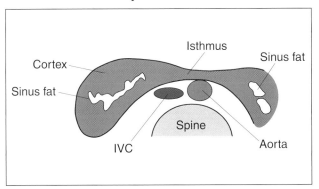

1d. Duplex kidney

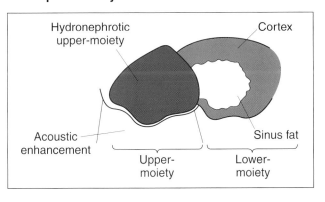

Scan image

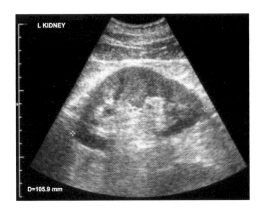

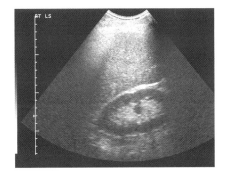

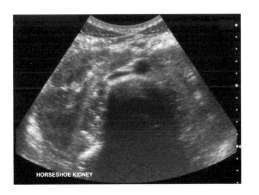

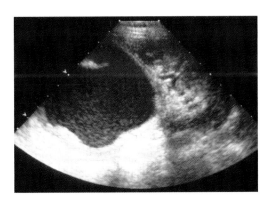

2. Simple renal cysts

These are a very common finding, increasing in frequency with age. They are most commonly located in the cortex.

Ultrasound features

- Smooth edge
- Thin wall
- Echo-free contents (may contain a few fine septations)
- Postacoustic enhancement

3. Adult polycystic kidney disease (PCKD)

In this autosomal dominant condition, the kidneys contain multiple numbers of cysts, which slowly enlarge, causing cortical thinning and progressive renal failure. The cysts may be visible on ultrasound by the second decade but usually remain asymptomatic until mid-40s.

Ultrasound features

- The kidneys are enlarged, with an undulating surface
- They contain multiple cysts of varying sizes
- The cysts are typically simple but some may have a more complex appearance due to internal haemorrhage

Look for associated cysts in the liver (50%), pancreas (10%) and spleen (rare).

4. Renal stones (nephrolithiasis)

Calcium containing stones are the most common type. Patients are often asymptomatic, but may suffer recurrent urinary tract infections or bouts of renal colic.

Ultrasound features

- Echo-bright focus that casts a distal acoustic shadow
- May be difficult to detect if obscured by renal sinus echoes
- If a stone has caused ureteric obstruction then hydronephrosis may be seen

Hint: Always measure the size of any stones and note their location.
Hint: Increasing the frequency and reducing the overall gain makes stone detection easier.

What to look for

Scan image

2. Simple renal cyst

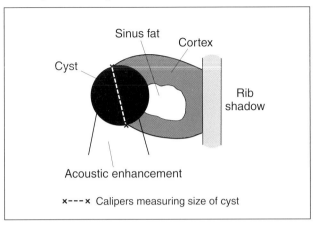

Sinus fat · Cortex · Cyst · Rib shadow · Acoustic enhancement

x---x Calipers measuring size of cyst

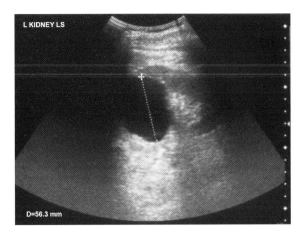

3. Adult PCKD

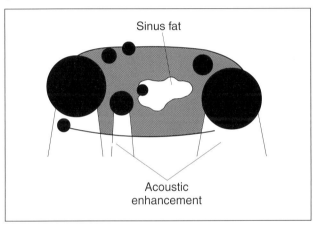

Sinus fat · Acoustic enhancement

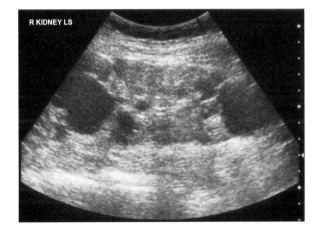

4. Renal stones

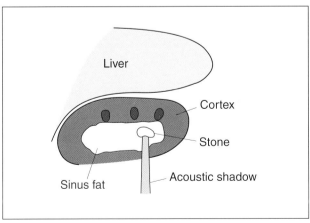

Liver · Cortex · Stone · Acoustic shadow · Sinus fat

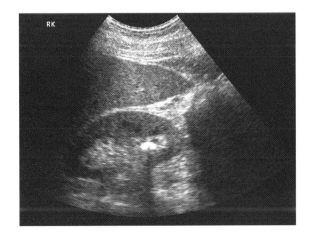

5. Hydronephrosis

This is obstructive dilation of the collecting system; most commonly caused by a stone, tumour or blood clot. It can be graded as follows:

(a) Mild

There is separation of renal sinus echoes – the 'split sinus' sign. This should be differentiated from back-pressure effects of a full bladder by rescanning the patient after they have voided; the system should decompress within a few minutes. It should also be differentiated from prominent renal vessels by using colour Doppler.

(b) Moderate

The pelvis and calyces are swollen, but there is no loss of cortical thickness.

(c) Severe

The system is grossly swollen, with loss of sinus fat echoes and cortical thinning.

What to look for

5a. Mild hydronephrosis

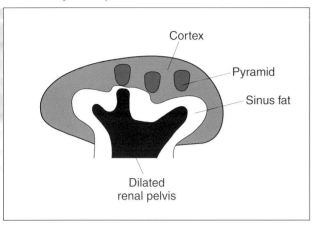

Scan image

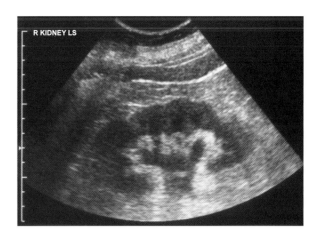

5b. Moderate hydronephrosis

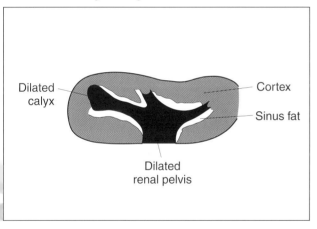

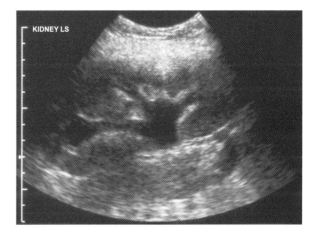

5c. Severe hydronephrosis

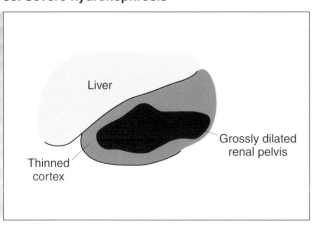

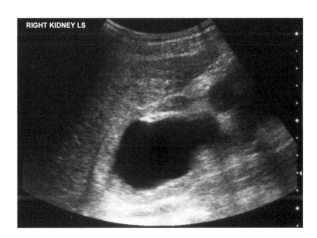

6. Angiomyolipoma

This is a benign mixed tumour of blood vessels, muscle and fat. It tends to enlarge with age and is more common in females.

Ultrasound features

- Cortical-based lesion
- Usually a small (<2 cm) sharply defined echo-bright mass
- One-third will cast a postacoustic shadow
- Multiple bilateral lesions may be seen in tuberous sclerosis patients

Larger angiomyolipomas (>3 cm) can mimic the appearance of a small renal cell carcinoma and also have a recognized risk of spontaneous haemorrhage (especially if >4 cm); they are therefore kept under ultrasound review.

7. Renal cell carcinoma (RCC)

This is the most common renal malignancy in adults.

Ultrasound features

- Mass lesion, usually of mixed echogenicity, often causing bulging of the renal contour
- Small tumours can be echo-bright and look similar to angiomyolipomas

It is important to assess the renal vein and inferior vena cava for tumour thrombus. The other kidney should also be inspected carefully, as 5% are bilateral!

8. Renal artery stenosis (RAS)

This presents clinically as resistant hypertension. The majority of cases are caused by atherosclerosis, which tends to involve the proximal portion of the MRA. Rarely, it is due to fibromuscular dysplasia, which affects the MRA more distally. RAS is thought to be clinically significant only if the stenosis is >70%.

Ultrasound features

- Unilateral small kidney (>2 cm size difference)
- Direct MRA spectral Doppler shows a peak-systolic velocity >180 cm/s or a ratio to peak-systolic aortic velocity >3.5
- Interlobar artery spectral Doppler shows loss of the normal sharp systolic upstroke. It has a dampened, rounded 'parvus tardus' waveform with acceleration time (AT) >0.07 s and more specifically >0.12 s.

What to look for	*Scan image*

6. Angiomyolipoma

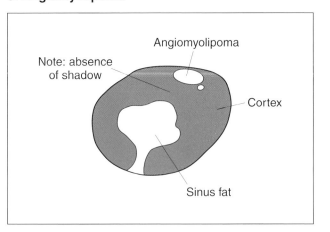

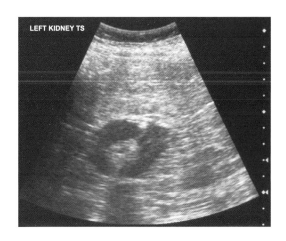

7. RCC

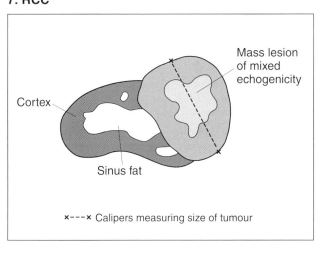

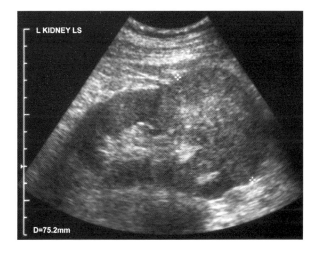

8. RAS

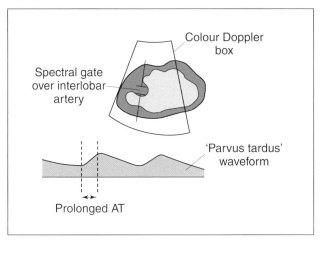

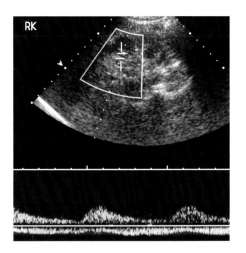

9. Renal failure

(a) Acute renal failure

There is significant deterioration of renal function over hours–days.
- **Prerenal**: caused by hypoperfusion.
- **Renal**: causes include acute glomerulonephritis and acute tubular necrosis (e.g. contrast reaction).
- **Postrenal**: due to outflow obstruction (e.g. ovarian malignancy, ureteric stone).

Ultrasound features

Prerenal/renal
- Kidneys are usually of normal size
- Renal cortex may be echo-bright and/or swollen
- Pyramids can appear prominent: 'punched-out pyramids' sign
- Interlobar artery RI is usually raised

Postrenal
- Look for hydronephrosis (see earlier)

(b) Chronic renal failure

There is long-standing loss of renal function over months–years. Causes include chronic glomerulonephritis and diabetic/hypertensive nephropathy.

Ultrasound features
- Kidneys are small (it may be impossible to find them)
- Renal cortex is thinned and echo-bright

10. Renal infarct

This is a severe ischaemic event causing death of a segment of renal parenchyma. Causes include:
- embolism: infective endocarditis, post-myocardial infarction mural thrombus
- thrombosis: vasculitis, sickle cell disease crisis
- trauma: causing injury to the main renal artery

Ultrasound features
- Echo-bright wedge-shaped cortical defect

What to look for

9a. Acute renal failure

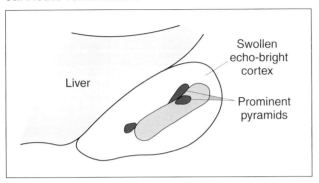

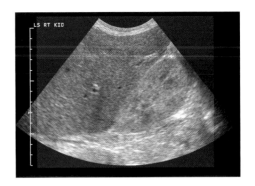

9b. Chronic renal failure

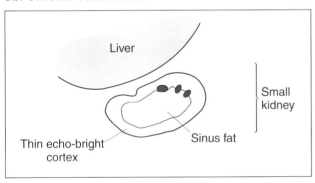

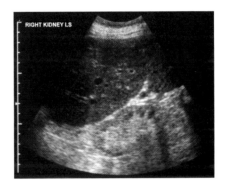

10. Renal infarct

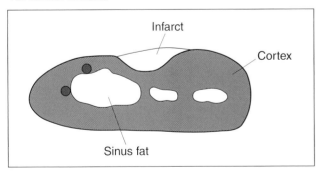

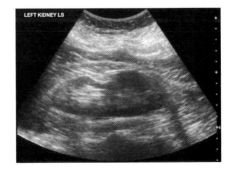

11. Bladder wall thickening

The bladder needs to be well-distended for accurate assessment. Wall thickness >5 mm is abnormal. Chronic bacterial cystitis is a common cause of generalized thickening.

A focal thickening may be due to a bladder cancer (e.g. TCC) and must be distinguished from a haematoma – cancers will not move on patient re-positioning and may display internal blood flow with colour Doppler.

12. Ureterocele

This is a cystic dilation of the distal ureter at its bladder insertion. There is a strong association with duplex kidneys, where the ureter draining the upper-moiety tends to be the one involved. Ureteroceles can cause ureteric obstruction, and stones may form within them.

Ultrasound features
- Thin-walled cystic projection at the site of ureteric insertion
- Always look for any associated obstruction (hydroureter or hydronephrosis)

What to look for

11a. Bladder wall thickening

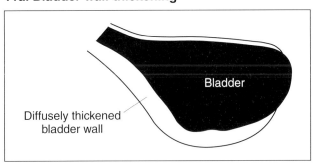

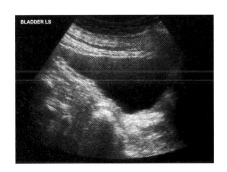

11b. Bladder carcinoma

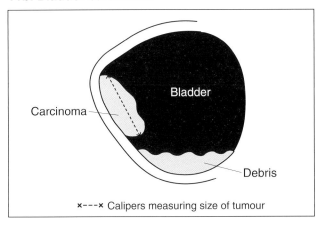

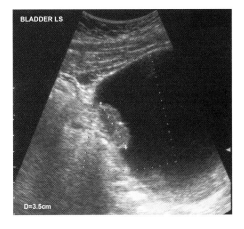

12. Ureterocele

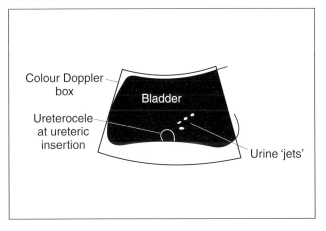

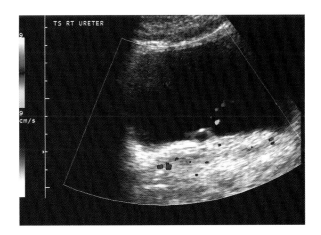

13. Transplant kidney fluid collections

Collections of blood, lymph and urine around the transplant are very common in the postoperative period. Most are incidental findings, and resolve spontaneously. However, occasionally they can be large and compress the graft, impairing its function. These may then need drainage.

Ultrasound features

Lymphocele
- Commonest collection
- Occurs weeks to months postoperation
- Seen as an echo-free area which classically has internal septations

Haematoma
- Occurs immediately postoperation
- In early stages, seen as an echo-free area
- May later contain echo-bright fibrin strands

Urinoma
- Uncommon collection
- Occurs early postoperation
- Seen as an echo-free area

Ultrasound cannot usually distinguish between these different collections; however, it has a role to play in monitoring their regression. Rarely, a collection may become infected, leading to abscess formation.

14. Transplant rejection (acute)

This is mediated via cellular immunity. It occurs most commonly during the first month postoperation. The patient is systemically unwell, with a tender swollen graft.

Ultrasound features
- Swollen kidney
- Echo-bright renal cortex
- Reduced brightness of renal sinus fat
- Interlobar artery spectral Doppler RI > 0.7

These features are also seen in acute tubular necrosis and cyclosporin toxicity, and they should be considered in conjunction with the patient history. Serial RI values may help but often a biopsy is needed to establish the diagnosis.

What to look for

Scan image

13a. Post-transplant lymphocele

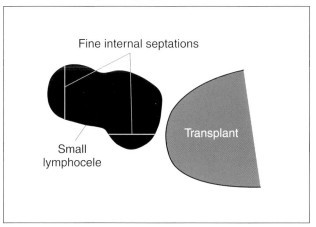

Fine internal septations

Transplant

Small
lymphocele

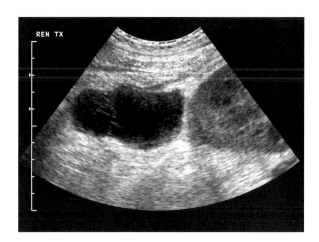

13b. Post-transplant urinoma

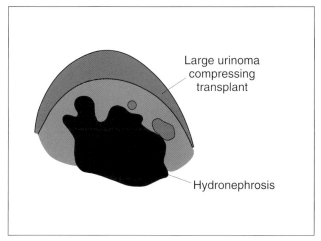

Large urinoma
compressing
transplant

Hydronephrosis

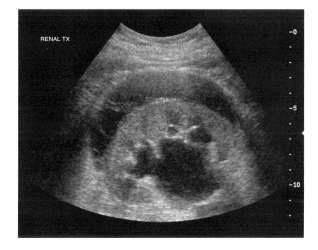

14. Transplant rejection (acute)

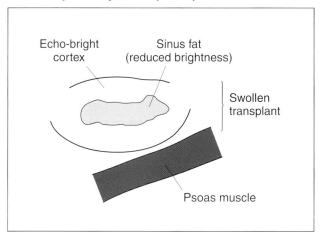

Echo-bright
cortex

Sinus fat
(reduced brightness)

Swollen
transplant

Psoas muscle

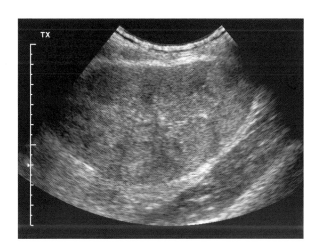

15. Transplant kidney main renal vein (MRV) thrombosis

This is a rare, but serious, early complication. The patient will be oliguric, with a tender, swollen graft.

Ultrasound features

• Swollen kidney with subcapsular fluid collections
• Reduced cortical perfusion
• Note absence of flow in the MRV
• Look for the characteristic MRA waveform, which shows reverse end-diastolic flow

The transplant is non-viable, and must be removed.

What to look for

15. Transplant kidney MRV thrombosis

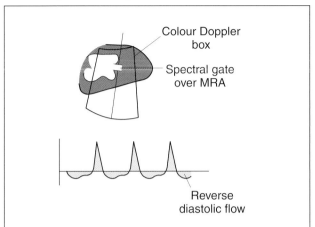

Colour Doppler box

Spectral gate over MRA

Reverse diastolic flow

Scan image

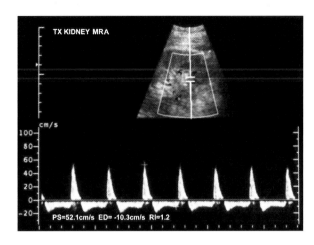

TX KIDNEY MRA

cm/s

100—
80—
60—
40—
20—
0—
-20—

PS=52.1cm/s ED= -10.3cm/s RI=1.2

5

Abdominal aorta

ANATOMY

Anterior view of abdominal aorta

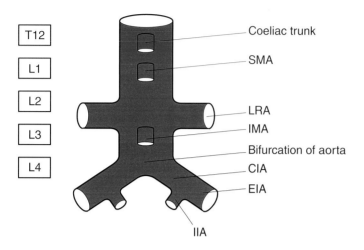

T12	Coeliac trunk
L1	SMA
L2	LRA
L3	IMA
L4	Bifurcation of aorta
	CIA
	EIA
	IIA

Transverse section of renal arteries and aorta

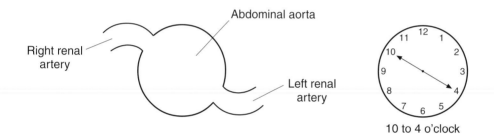

Abdominal aorta

Right renal artery

Left renal artery

10 to 4 o'clock

In TS section, the renal arteries are seen to branch off the aorta at the 10 to 4 o'clock positions.

Key points

1. The main branches of the aorta exit at the following vertebral levels:

Artery	Approximate vertebral level
Coeliac trunk	T12
SMA	L1
Renal arteries	L2/3
IMA	L3
Bifurcation of aorta	L4

2. Normal diameter of abdominal aorta <2 cm.
3. Normal diameter of common iliac arteries <1 cm.

PERFORMING THE SCAN

- **Patient position**: Supine.
- **Preparation**: Nil by mouth for 8 hours.
- **Probe**: Low-frequency (3–5 MHz) curvilinear.
- **Machine**: Select the abdomen preset mode. Set the focus at the posterior wall of the aorta. Use tissue harmonics if the SNR is poor or with obese patients.
- **Method**: Start at the upper abdomen and scan caudally in at least two planes. Acquire more than one representative image for each step if pathology is found.

Probe position

Instructions

1. TS: upper abdominal aorta

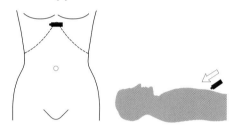

- Place the probe just inferior to the xiphisternum and angle it cranially. Look for the 'seagull sign' of the coeliac trunk at T12 level. The body of the 'seagull' is the coeliac trunk and the wings are the hepatic and splenic arteries branching off.
- Acquire representative image(s).

2. TS: aorta

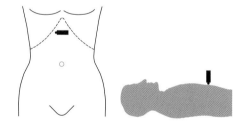

- Now angle the probe so that it is perpendicular to the abdomen and scan caudally, following the course of the aorta until it bifurcates. Look for any irregularities in the vessel wall.
- Measure the maximum AP diameter in TS of the suprarenal aorta and infrarenal aorta.
- The renal arteries are difficult to visualize directly. To locate the region of the renal arteries, first look for the 'tadpole sign' of the portal confluence/splenic vein, then look posterior to this to find the SMA. The renal arteries arise 1 cm caudal to the SMA origin.
- Acquire representative image(s).

3. Colour Doppler TS: aorta

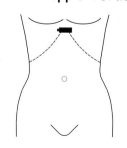

- Place the probe just inferior to the xiphisternum again. Turn on colour Doppler and place the colour box over the aorta.
- Optimize the colour signal: adjust the colour gain and focus position, narrow the sector width, reduce the colour box size, and set the PRF at high and the filter at medium.
- Scan caudally, following the course of the aorta until it bifurcates. Look for any filling defects.
- Acquire representative image(s).

What to look for

Scan image

1.

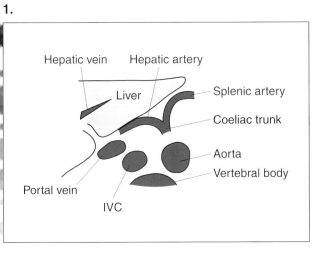

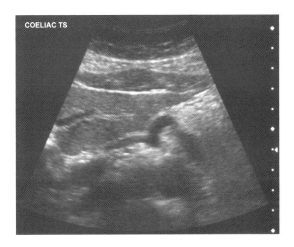

2.

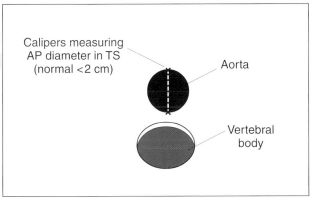

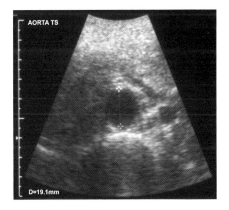

3.

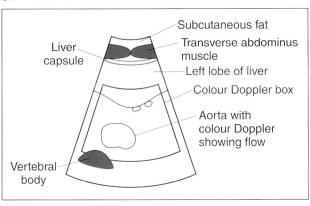

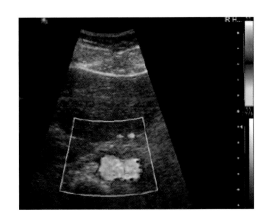

Probe position	**Instructions**

4. LS: aorta

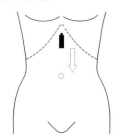

- Return to the xiphisternum and locate the upper abdominal aorta in TS as in Step 1.
- Rotate the probe through 90° clockwise so that the aorta is now imaged in LS.
- Follow the course of the aorta caudally in LS until it bifurcates. Look for any vessel wall irregularities.
- Look specifically for the origin of the SMA: just posterior to this the LRV should be visible, and it should be possible to describe any anomalies in relation to the renal vessels. The distance from the SMA to any aneurysm should be measured and documented.
- If there is difficulty in following the aorta in LS, try a coronal view instead – i.e. place the probe in the left flank and angle it towards the vertebral column.
- Acquire representative image(s).

5. Colour Doppler LS: aorta

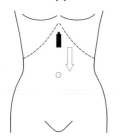

- Now turn on colour Doppler and place the colour box over the aorta.
- Optimize the colour signal: adjust the gain and focus position, narrow the FOV, reduce the colour box size, and set the PRF at high and the filter at medium. Doppler angle should be 0°–60° to demonstrate flow.
- Repeat Step 4, looking for any filling defects.
- Acquire representative image(s).

6. Common iliac arteries

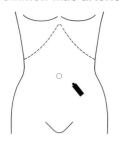

- Turn off colour Doppler. Place the probe over the bifurcation of the aorta in TS, then follow each CIA caudally as far as possible, looking for any vessel wall irregularities.
- Measure the maximum AP diameter of each CIA in TS but if this proves too difficult measure approximately in LS.
- Turn on colour Doppler and repeat this step, looking for any filling defects.
- Return the probe to the bifurcation of the aorta in TS. Rotate the probe through 90° clockwise and now scan each CIA in LS with and without colour Doppler.
- Acquire representative image(s).

What to look for   **Scan image**

4.

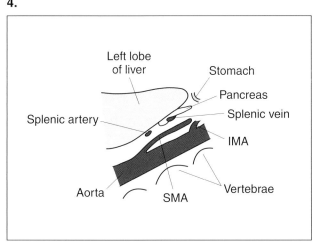

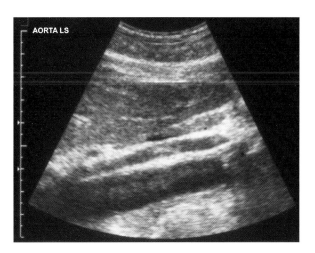

5.

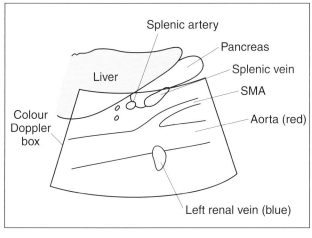

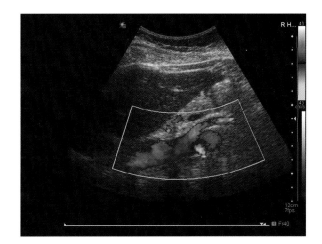

6.

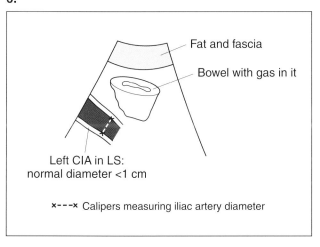

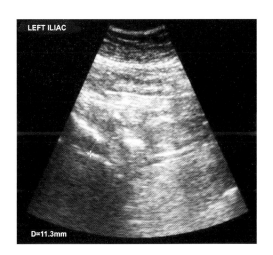

ABDOMINAL AORTA: COMMON PATHOLOGY

1. Atheromatous plaques

Atherosclerosis is a disease of large and medium-sized muscular arteries. It is characterized by the accumulation of lipids, calcium and cellular debris within the intima of the vessel wall, forming atheromatous plaques. These plaques result in luminal obstruction, abnormalities of blood flow and diminished oxygen supply to target organs. The major risk factors are smoking, hypercholesterolaemia, diabetes and hypertension.

Ultrasound features
- Localized irregular thickening of the vessel wall (measure in TS and LS)
- The echogenicity of the plaque depends on its contents:
  - echo-poor: blood- or lipid-filled = increased risk of rupture
  - echo-bright: calcified = more benign
- Filling defects with colour Doppler
- Classify using the Gray–Weale classification

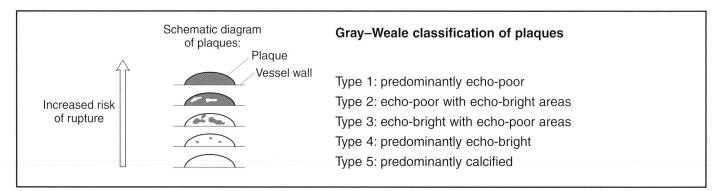

Schematic diagram of plaques:
Plaque
Vessel wall
Increased risk of rupture

Gray–Weale classification of plaques

Type 1: predominantly echo-poor

Type 2: echo-poor with echo-bright areas

Type 3: echo-bright with echo-poor areas

Type 4: predominantly echo-bright

Type 5: predominantly calcified

2. Aneurysm

An aneurysm is a localized dilation of an artery by at least 50% (<50% = ectasia) compared with the normal diameter of the vessel. Aneurysms occur in 5% of patients >65 years old. Major risk factors are atherosclerosis, age and inflammation (e.g. malignancy, syphilis). Aneurysms <5.5 cm are usually monitored with ultrasound scan every 6 months.

Ultrasound features
- Localized dilation of artery: measure AP diameter in TS from outer wall to outer wall
- Usually aneurysms are infrarenal
- Filling defects with colour Doppler

Diameter (cm)	Description	Risk of rupture	Action
<2	Normal		Nil
2.5–2.9	Ectatic		Monitor 6 monthly
3–5.4	Low-risk aneurysm	1% per year	Monitor 6 monthly
>5.5	High-risk aneurysm	5% per year	Refer to vascular team on the same day
>7	Aneurysm emergency!	>25% per year	Refer to vascular team IMMEDIATELY

Note: If the patient has any symptoms related to the aneurysm – e.g. abdominal/back pain, collapse, etc. (regardless of the size of the aneurysm) – discuss with the vascular team on the same day.

What to look for

1. Atheromatous plaques

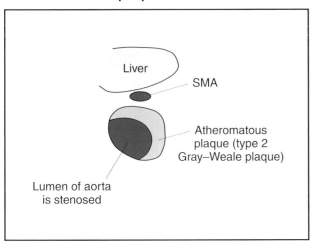

Scan image

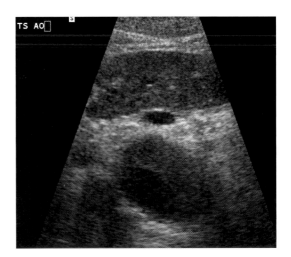

2a. Aneurysmal aorta

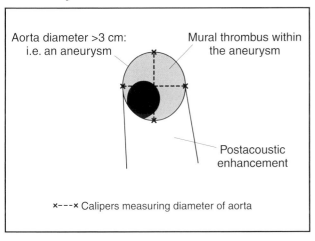

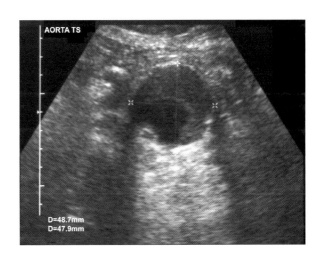

2b. Ectactic aorta

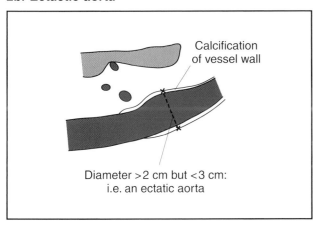

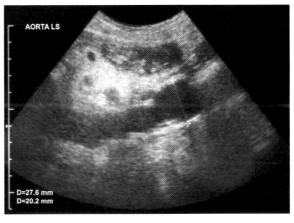

6

Liver transplant

PRETRANSPLANT: INDICATIONS FOR SCAN

There are two groups of patients upon whom the preoperative liver transplant protocol should be performed:

1. Those who are known to have chronic liver disease and are being considered for the transplant waiting list.
2. Those who have evidence of chronic liver disease on ultrasound – e.g. a cirrhotic liver, alcoholic liver disease, ascites or splenomegaly – and may potentially require a transplant in the future.

The indications for liver transplantation are as follows:

1. Cirrhosis from chronic liver disease:
    *   hepatitis
    *   alcoholic liver disease
    *   primary biliary cirrhosis
    *   primary sclerosing cholangitis
    *   Wilson's disease
    *   haemochromatosis
    *   Budd–Chiari syndrome
2. Fulminant hepatic failure – e.g. paracetamol overdose or acute hepatitis.
3. Congenital liver failure:
    *   polycystic disease
    *   Caroli's disease
4. Hepatocellular carcinoma (HCC).

PRETRANSPLANT: MAIN AIMS OF SCAN

1. Confirm the initial diagnosis (if there is one).
2. Assess vessel patency.
3. Assess any associated complications.
4. Assess any contraindications to transplant:
   - extrahepatic malignancy
   - systemic sepsis
   - cholangiocarcinoma
   - porto–superior mesenteric vein thrombosis
   - HCC >5 cm or >3 HCC tumours

PRETRANSPLANT: PERFORMING THE SCAN

- **Patient position**: Supine.
- **Preparation**: Clear fluid only for 8 hours.
- **Probe**: Low-frequency (3–5 MHz) curvilinear.
- **Machine**: Select abdomen preset mode.
- **Method**: (a) Full abdomen scan (see abdomen protocol), looking specifically for cirrhosis, ascites, splenomegaly and varices.
  (b) Perform Doppler examination of hepatic artery, hepatic veins, portal vein, splenic vein and inferior vena cava.

Probe position	*Instructions*
1. Liver 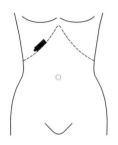	<ul><li>Place the probe in the RUQ and scan through the liver in at least two planes.</li><li>It is often difficult to clearly image a shrunken cirrhotic liver. Therefore ask the patient to take deep breaths in as the probe is angled caudally under the subcostal margin. If there is still difficulty imaging the liver, try an intercostal approach.</li><li>Examine the liver, taking note of: – any focal lesions, metastases, HCC? – echogenicity: diffuse and focal – echotexture: coarse? – size: is it shrunken and cirrhotic? – surface: is it nodular or smooth? – ducts: are they dilated?</li><li>Examine the subphrenic and subhepatic spaces. Look specifically for ascites.</li><li>Acquire representative images.</li></ul>
2. Complete abdomen protocol scan	<ul><li>See Chapter 3 for details.</li><li>Pay particular attention to the following: – CBD: measure diameter – spleen: is there splenomegaly? – any contraindications to transplant?</li><li>Acquire representative images.</li></ul>

What to look for

1.

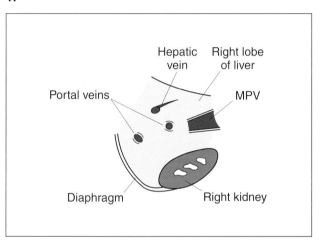

Scan image

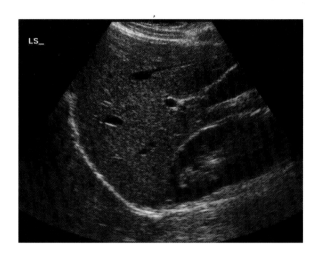

2.

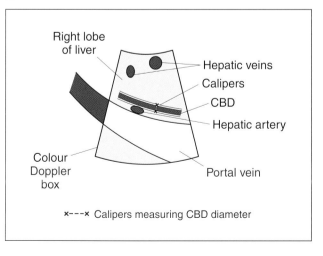

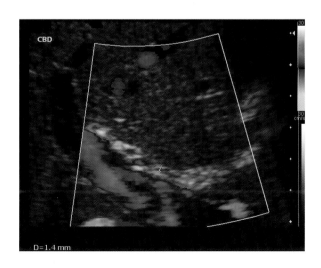

Probe position	Instructions

3. Main hepatic artery spectral Doppler

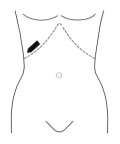

- Place the probe in the RUQ intercostally. The position varies between patients, but try the 11th ICS AAL or MCL. Find the portal vein and then look anterior to it to visualize the MHA.
- Turn on colour Doppler. Optimize the colour signal: adjust the colour gain and focus position, narrow the FOV, reduce the colour box size, and set the PRF at medium and the filter at medium.
- Take note of flow in the hepatic artery. If no flow is detected, turn up the colour gain and reduce the PRF scale. If still no flow is detected, the hepatic artery may be occluded.
- If flow is detected, turn on spectral Doppler and place the gate over the hepatic artery, acquiring a trace. Optimize the waveform by adjusting the gate size and ensuring a beam-flow angle of $0°–60°$.
  Hint: Ask the patient to breathe gently or hold their breath to aid measurement.
- Select the calculation package. Calculate the acceleration time (AT) via the interval from end-diastole to the *first* peak of the systolic upstroke. Calculate the resistance index (RI) via the peak-systolic value S and the trough diastolic value D: $RI = (S − D)/S$.
- Normal values are RI >0.5 and AT <0.08 s.
- Acquire representative image(s).

4. Main portal vein spectral Doppler

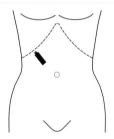

- Find the portal vein by placing the probe perpendicular to the right costal margin MCL.
- Turn on colour Doppler and assess patency.
- Turn on spectral Doppler and place the gate over the portal vein, acquiring a trace. Optimize the waveform by adjusting the gate size and ensuring a beam-flow angle of $60°$. Measure the peak velocity and record the direction and character of flow.
- Normal peak velocity = 16–40 cm/s.
- Normal direction: hepatopetal.
- Normal character: alters with respiration; may have transmitted pulsation from IVC in a slim patient.
- Acquire representative image(s).

What to look for

Scan image

3.

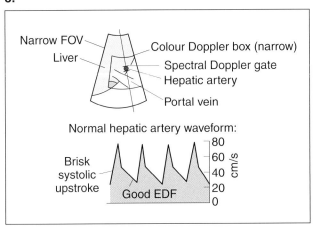

Normal hepatic artery waveform:

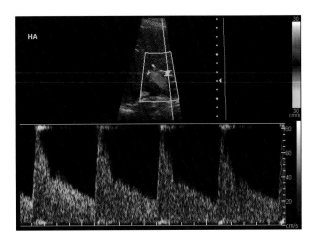

4.

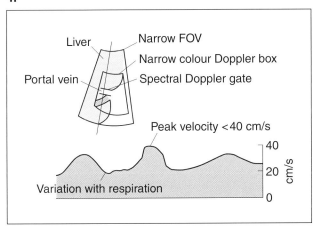

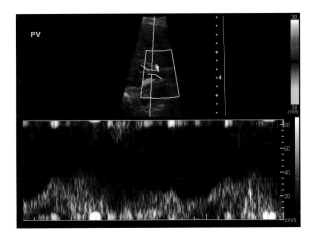

Probe position	**Instructions**

5. Hepatic veins spectral Doppler

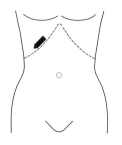

- To examine the hepatic veins, place the probe parallel to the right costal margin and angle it caudally under the costal margin as the patient inspires. If there is difficulty finding the hepatic veins, try an intercostal approach.
- Turn on colour Doppler and optimize the colour signal as described in Step 1.
- Assess the patency of all three hepatic veins.
- Turn on spectral Doppler and place the gate over a hepatic vein, acquiring a trace. Optimize the waveform by adjusting the gate size.
- The normal waveform is a classical triphasic pattern and varies with respiration.
- Acquire representative image(s).

6. IVC spectral Doppler

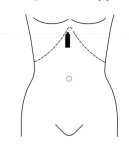

- To image the IVC, place the probe LS inferior to the xiphisternum and just right of the midine.
- Alternatively, place the probe in the right MCL and angle it towards the left flank.
- Turn on colour Doppler to assess patency.
- Turn on spectral Doppler and place the gate over the IVC, acquiring a trace. Optimize the waveform by adjusting the gate size.
- Normal flow is pulsatile with reverse flow during right atrial systole; it varies with respiration.
- Acquire representative image(s).

7. Splenic vein spectral Doppler

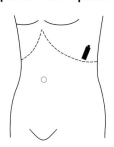

- Ask the patient to turn 45° onto the right side.
- Place the probe in the left 11th ICS AAL to image the spleen. Measure the spleen length.
- Turn on colour Doppler and locate the splenic vein. Is it patent? Are there any varices? Follow the course of the splenic vein posterior to the pancreas.
- Turn on spectral Doppler and place the gate over the splenic vein, acquiring a trace. Optimize the waveform by adjusting the gate size and ensuring a beam-flow angle of 0°–60°.
- Normal flow is hepatopetal/away from the probe and varies with respiration.
- Acquire representative image(s).

What to look for

5.

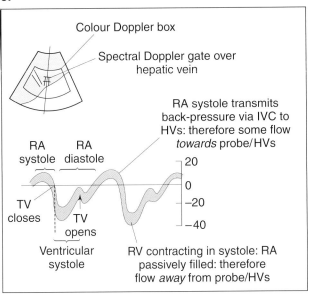

Colour Doppler box

Spectral Doppler gate over hepatic vein

RA systole transmits back-pressure via IVC to HVs: therefore some flow *towards* probe/HVs

RA systole   RA diastole

TV closes

TV opens

Ventricular systole

RV contracting in systole: RA passively filled: therefore flow *away* from probe/HVs

20
0
−20
−40

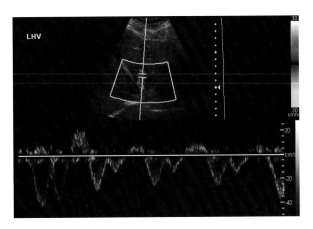

6.

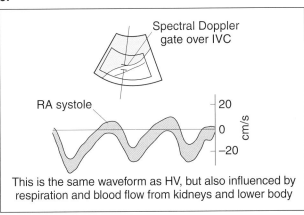

Spectral Doppler gate over IVC

RA systole

20
0   cm/s
−20

This is the same waveform as HV, but also influenced by respiration and blood flow from kidneys and lower body

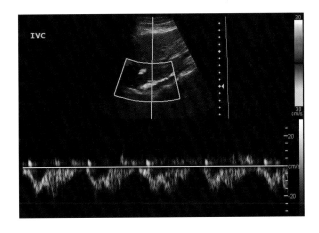

7.

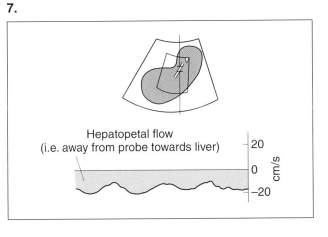

Hepatopetal flow (i.e. away from probe towards liver)

20
0   cm/s
−20

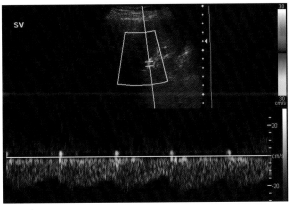

PRETRANSPLANT: PATHOLOGY

Refer also to the hepatobiliary pathology section in Chapter 3.

1. Portal hypertension

Increased pressure in the portal venous system results in blood from the gut bypassing the liver via collateral veins. These veins then dilate and form varices. The most common causes are cirrhosis, alcoholic hepatitis and portal vein thrombosis.

Ultrasound features

• Portal vein flow varies with severity of hypertension:

Degree of portal hypertension	Spectral Doppler waveform
Very mild	Loss of variation with respiration
Mild	Slowed peak velocity, i.e. <10 cm/s
Moderate	Balanced, i.e. forward and reverse flow together
Severe	Reversed flow
Complete occlusion	No flow

• Hepatic artery may show increased flow (compensating for reduced flow into liver from portal vein)
• Associated features:
  – ascites
  – varices
  – splenomegaly
  – recanalized umbilical vein

2. Portal vein thrombosis

Thrombosis may cause complete or partial occlusion of the vein. The most common causes are cirrhosis, pancreatitis and gastrointestinal malignancy. HCC may result in tumour thrombus in the portal vein, and arterial flow may be seen within the portal vein due to neo-angiogenesis (with colour Doppler).

Two to three weeks after a portal vein is thrombosed, a mass of tortuous vessels may form at the porta hepatis. This is called cavernous transformation and may be mistaken for biliary dilation unless colour and spectral Doppler are used to identify flow in the vessels.

Ultrasound features

• Fresh thrombus: echo-free
• >24-hour-old thrombus: low-level echoes
• Cavernous transformation (see above)
• Colour Doppler: a filling defect if thrombosis causes stenosis
• Colour Doppler: no flow if the thrombosis causes occlusion
• Spectral Doppler: increased velocity at stenosis site

What to look for	*Scan image*

1a. Portal hypertension (mild/moderate)

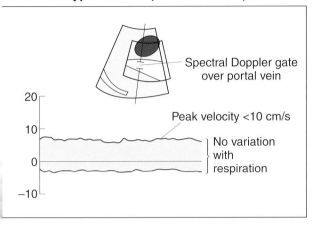

Spectral Doppler gate over portal vein

Peak velocity <10 cm/s

No variation with respiration

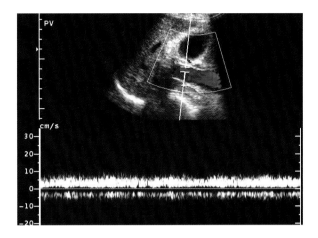

1b. Portal hypertension (severe)

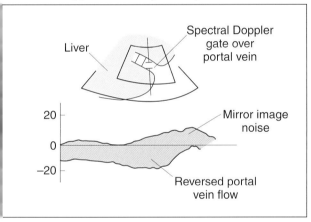

Liver

Spectral Doppler gate over portal vein

Mirror image noise

Reversed portal vein flow

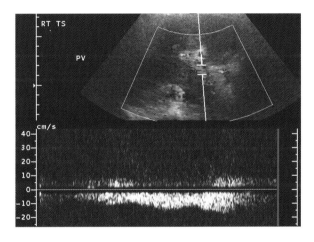

2. Portal vein thrombosis

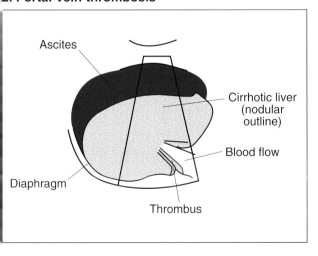

Ascites

Cirrhotic liver (nodular outline)

Blood flow

Diaphragm

Thrombus

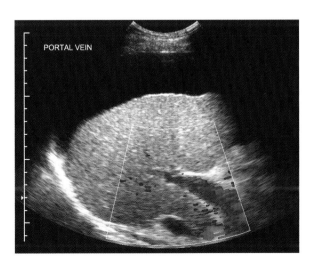

3. Budd–Chiari syndrome

This is obstruction of hepatic veins by thrombus, tumour or a congenital fibrous web. The risk factors include pregnancy, malignancy, coagulation disorders and the oral contraceptive pill. In >50% of cases, it is idiopathic. Note that the same features may arise from IVC thrombosis.

Ultrasound features
• Acute stage: hepatomegaly
• Chronic stage: cirrhosis, regenerative nodules, enlargement of caudate lobe
• Splenomegaly
• Ascites
• Colour Doppler:
  – intrahepatic collaterals
  – reversed/no flow in hepatic veins, with or without stenotic segments
  – vein–vein shunting from one vein to another
• Spectral Doppler:
  – loss of normal hepatic vein triphasic waveform
  – waveform may be absent, turbulent, reversed or monophasic
  – reversed flow in IVC

Appendix: Explanation of triphasic hepatic vein waveform

The hepatic vein waveform corresponds to the venous pressure in the right atrium. The pressure from the right atrium is transmitted to the hepatic veins via the IVC.

1. During atrial systole, there is back-pressure to the IVC and hepatic veins. The hepatic flow is towards the probe, i.e. hepatopetal and away from the heart.
2. The tricuspid valve then closes and the right ventricle contracts. During ventricular systole, the right atrium fills passively, and therefore the hepatic flow is towards the heart, i.e. hepatofugal.
3. As the right atrium fills with blood, the pressure increases, resulting in a slower rate of flow into the right atrium.
4. The tricuspid valve opens at the end of ventricular systole, the right atrial pressure drops slightly, and so the rate of flow into the right atrium increases again.
5. Blood passively fills the right ventricle during ventricular diastole, resulting in a pressure rise.
6. At the end of ventricular diastole, the atrium contracts, resulting again in a surge of pressure, which is transmitted to the hepatic vein waveform.

What to look for

3. Budd–Chiari syndrome

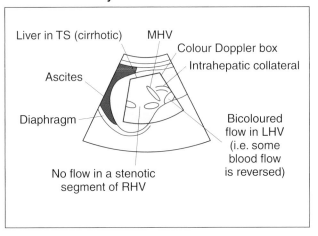

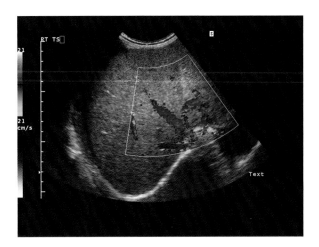

Appendix : Triphasic hepatic vein waveform

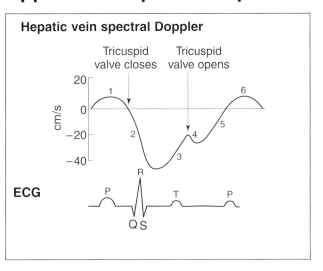

POST-TRANSPLANT: ANATOMY

The surgical procedure of a liver transplantation comprises:

1. A cholecystectomy.
2. An orthotopic transplant (i.e. the transplant liver is in the same anatomical position as the native organ), with five surgical anastomoses:
     (i) suprahepatic IVC
    (ii) infrahepatic IVC
    (iii) main portal vein
    (iv) hepatic artery
     (v) CBD (usually to a Roux bowel loop)

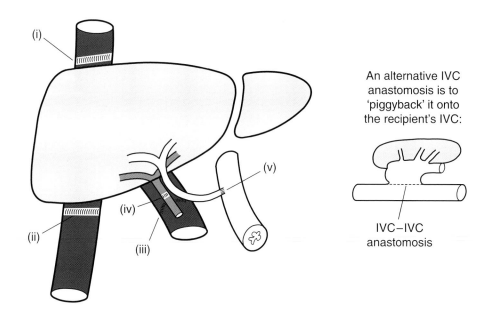

An alternative IVC anastomosis is to 'piggyback' it onto the recipient's IVC:

IVC–IVC anastomosis

POST-TRANSPLANT: MAIN AIMS OF THE SCAN

Assess for postoperative complications

- Anastomotic leaks/haematoma/stenosis/thrombosis
- Bile duct leaks/biloma/stenosis/stricture
- Infection/hepatic abscess

Assess for immunosuppression side-effects

- Undersuppressed: rejection
- Oversuppressed: renal impairment

POST-TRANSPLANT: PERFORMING THE SCAN

- **Patient position**: Supine.
- **Preparation**: None.
- **Probe**: Low-frequency (3–5 MHz) curvilinear *with a probe cover* (risk of cross-infection).
- **Machine**: Select abdomen preset mode.
- **Method**: Document date of transplant and number of days postoperation. Read the operation note if it is available. The post-transplant scan follows exactly the same steps as the pre-transplant scan. In both scans, a full abdomen protocol scan is completed and Doppler examinations of hepatic artery, hepatic veins, portal vein, splenic vein and inferior vena cava are performed. However, the likely pathologies are different and these are highlighted below. For further details of each step, refer to the pretransplant protocol. The salient points are summarized below.

Probe position	*Instructions*

Probe position

1. Liver

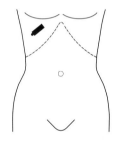

Instructions

- Place the probe in the RUQ and scan through the liver in TS and LS.
- In a patient who has had a recent transplant, there will be a 'Mercedes sign' surgical scar with dressings and possibly drains. This may interfere with the usual position of the probe for scanning. Therefore try angling the probe around the dressings or using an intercostal approach.
- Examine the liver parenchyma for:
  - any focal lesions
  - areas of infarction (hepatic artery insufficiency)
  - abscess
  - recurrence of HCC
  - PTLD
- Examine the subphrenic and subhepatic spaces, looking specifically for:
  - fluid collections, i.e. haematoma
  - biloma, abscess
  - ascites
  - pleural effusion (especially right)
- Note that there are no ultrasound features of rejection – a liver biopsy is needed for diagnosis.
- Acquire representative image(s).

What to look for

1.

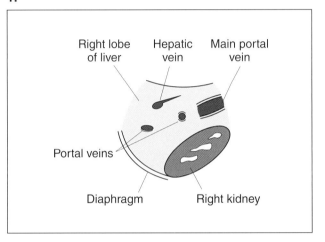

Scan image

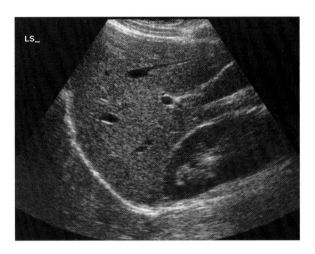

Probe position

Instructions

2. CBD

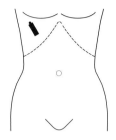

- Examine the CBD in two planes
- Measure its diameter:
    - Dilation can signify cholestasis and ascending infection.
    - Stenosis may signify anastomotic stricture or hepatic artery insufficiency.

    Hint: Remember that the gallbladder will have been removed during the transplant operation!
- Acquire representative image(s).

3. MHA spectral Doppler

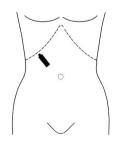

- Adults should be scanned on postoperative day 3. Before this, there may be false positives due to normal postsurgical features.
- Children should be scanned on postoperative day 1 because they are at a much higher risk of hepatic artery thrombosis.
- Place the probe in the RUQ intercostally. Find the portal vein and then look anterior to it to visualize the main hepatic artery.
- Turn on colour Doppler. Optimize the colour signal and take note of flow in the hepatic artery. Check both left and right branches.
- If no flow is detected, turn up the colour gain and reduce the PRF. If there is still no flow, try a lower-frequency probe. If, despite this, no flow is detected, the hepatic artery is likely to be occluded.
- If flow is detected, turn on spectral Doppler and place the gate over the hepatic artery, acquiring a trace.
- Within 48 hours postoperation, there may just be a small systolic spike with no EDF – this is not significant, and resolves within 48 hours.
- Acquire representative image(s).

4. MPV spectral Doppler

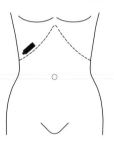

- Find the portal vein by placing the probe perpendicular to the right costal margin MCL.
- Turn on colour Doppler and assess patency.
- Turn on spectral Doppler and place the gate over the portal vein, acquiring a trace.
- Measure the peak velocity.
- Record the direction and character of flow.
- Postsurgery, the waveform usually appears turbulent around the anastomotic site. This is not significant unless it is associated with high peak velocities >100 cm/s.
- Acquire representative image(s).

What to look for	**Scan image**

2.

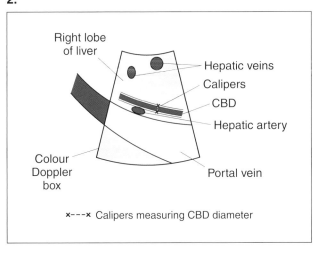

- Right lobe of liver
- Hepatic veins
- Calipers
- CBD
- Hepatic artery
- Colour Doppler box
- Portal vein

x---x Calipers measuring CBD diameter

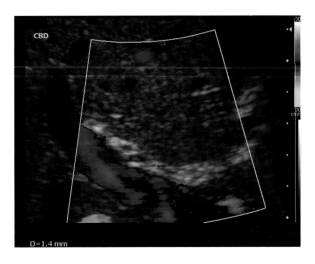

CBD

D=1.4 mm

3.

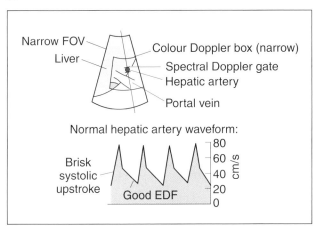

- Narrow FOV
- Liver
- Colour Doppler box (narrow)
- Spectral Doppler gate
- Hepatic artery
- Portal vein

Normal hepatic artery waveform:

Brisk systolic upstroke

Good EDF

80
60
40
20
0
cm/s

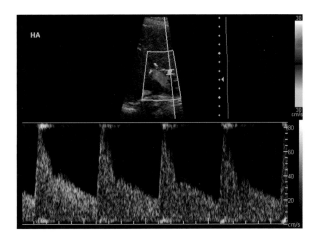

HA

4.

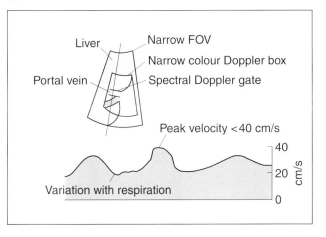

- Liver
- Narrow FOV
- Narrow colour Doppler box
- Spectral Doppler gate
- Portal vein

Peak velocity <40 cm/s

Variation with respiration

40
20
0
cm/s

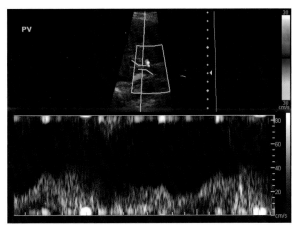

PV

Probe Position	**Instructions**

5. Hepatic veins spectral Doppler

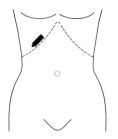

Repeat this step exactly as for the pretransplant scan. The technique is the same:

- Turn on colour Doppler and assess the patency of all three hepatic veins.
- Turn on spectral Doppler and place the gate over a hepatic vein, acquiring a trace.
- Acquire representative image(s).

6. IVC spectral Doppler

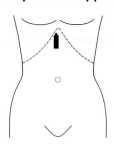

Repeat this step exactly as for the pretransplant scan. The technique is the same:

- Turn on colour Doppler to assess patency.
- Turn on spectral Doppler and place the gate over the IVC, acquiring a trace.
- Acquire representative image(s).

What to look for

Scan image

5.

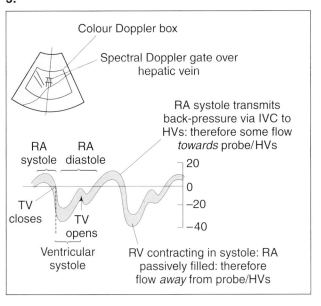

Colour Doppler box

Spectral Doppler gate over hepatic vein

RA systole transmits back-pressure via IVC to HVs: therefore some flow *towards* probe/HVs

RA systole

RA diastole

20
0
−20
−40

TV closes

TV opens

Ventricular systole

RV contracting in systole: RA passively filled: therefore flow *away* from probe/HVs

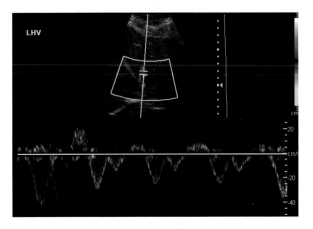

6.

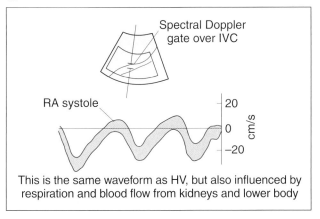

Spectral Doppler gate over IVC

RA systole

20
0
−20

cm/s

This is the same waveform as HV, but also influenced by respiration and blood flow from kidneys and lower body

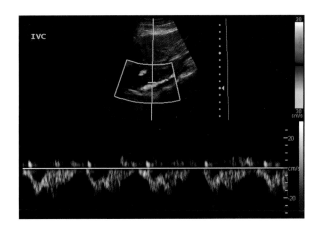

7. Splenic vein spectral Doppler

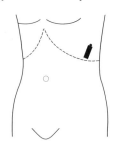

- Ask the patient to turn 45° onto the right side.
- Measure the spleen length. Note that if the spleen was enlarged prior to surgery then it will remain so in the early postoperative phase.
- Turn on colour Doppler and locate the splenic vein. Is the vein patent? Are there any varices? Note that varices may still be present in the initial postoperative phase.
- Turn on spectral Doppler and place the gate over the splenic vein, acquiring a trace.
- Acquire representative image(s).

8. Kidneys

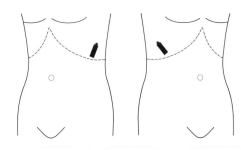

- Scan through both kidneys in two planes as for the abdominal ultrasound protocol.
- Look specifically for any evidence of renal impairment (a side-effect of the immunosuppressive drugs or due to intraoperative hypotension):
  - swollen enlarged kidneys
  - echo-bright cortex
- Acquire representative image(s).

7.

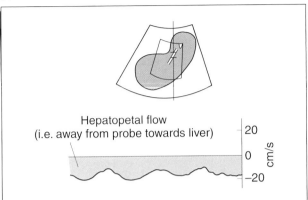

Hepatopetal flow
(i.e. away from probe towards liver)

20
0   cm/s
−20

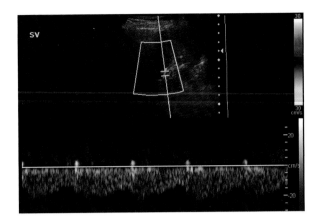

8.

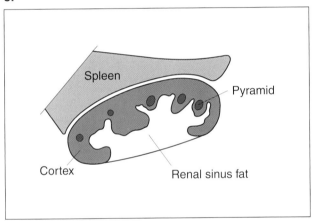

Spleen

Pyramid

Cortex

Renal sinus fat

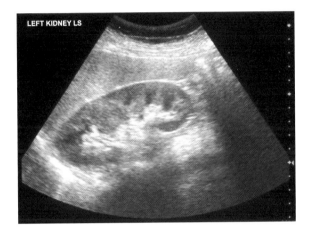

POST-TRANSPLANT: PATHOLOGY

1. Post-transplant collection

The main differential is between a haematoma and a biloma:

Haematoma

Most transplants have an immediate postoperative haematoma, usually in the gallbladder fossa. This is usually due to the trauma of surgery. If the patient is asymptomatic, no action is required. Beware a painful or rapidy enlarging haematoma – this may represent a vascular anastomotic leak, and requires further investigation.

Ultrasound features
- In early stages, seen as an echo-free area
- May later contain echo-bright fibrin strands
- Adjacent to liver and often posterior to the right lobe

Biloma

This is a collection of bile due to a bile duct anastomotic leak. It may lead to peritonitis. Bilomas usually occur in the first 2 months postoperation.

Ultrasound features
- Echo-poor collection
- May have internal echoes if sludge forms
- Occurs adjacent to the bile duct, either intra- or extraheptic

Note that ultrasound cannot differentiate reliably between blood, ascites, bile and pus.

2. Bile duct stricture

This occurs in 15% of transplant patients. It may occur many years after transplant. Stricture may be due either to the technical complications of the anastomosis or to diffuse injury secondary to hepatic artery thrombosis, rejection, etc.

Ultrasound features
- Narrowing of CBD
- Proximal intrahepatic duct dilatation

3. Post-transplant lymphoproliferative disorder (PTLD)

This occurs in 10% of transplant patients. It is a malignant disease with proliferation of B cells in lymph nodes and solid organs. There is an increased risk with high-dose immunosuppressive drugs and in patients with EBV. PTLD usually occurs within 1 year of transplant.

Ultrasound features
- Single or multiple focal echo-poor masses
- Masses may be vascular
- Can occur in liver allograft, bowel, kidneys, spleen
- Multiple sites of abdominal lymphadenopathy

What to look for

1. Haematoma

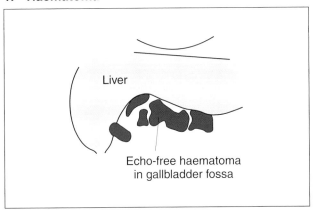

Scan image

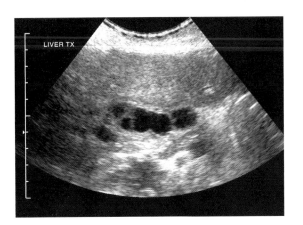

2. CBD stricture

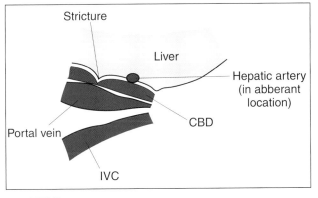

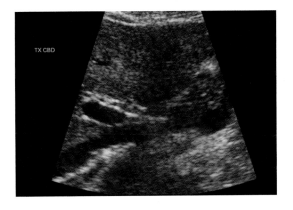

3. PTLD

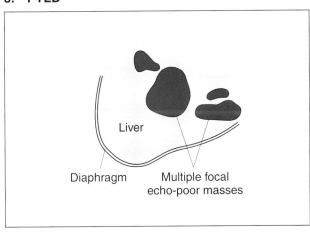

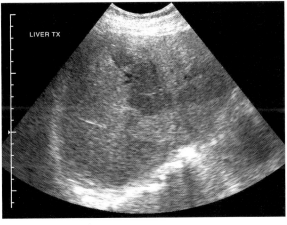

4. Hepatic artery stenosis

This occurs in approximately 5–10% of liver transplant patients. It usually occurs within the first few weeks after transplant. Hepatic artery stenosis can lead to hepatic infarction, abscess formation, bile duct necrosis and leakage. If liver abscess can be seen then there must be hepatic artery stenosis – the hepatic artery is the sole supply to the bile ducts.

Ultrasound features

- 'Parvus tardus' pattern distal to stenosis, i.e. slow systolic upstroke and increased EDF
- Acceleration time >0.08 s
- Resistance index <0.05

If this progresses, it may result in hepatic artery thrombosis.

5. Hepatic artery thrombosis

This occurs in approximately 5% of liver transplant patients. Complete occlusion of the hepatic artery is a surgical emergency because the artery provides oxygenation for the entire biliary system and therefore the liver quickly infarcts, with consequent biliary stasis, abscess formation and sepsis. The mortality rate without retransplantation is 75%.

Ultrasound features

- Absent colour Doppler flow
- Absent spectral Doppler waveform
- If collateral flow has developed, it may be seen as a 'parvus tardus' pattern

6. Hepatic vein thrombosis

Look specifically for hepatic vein thrombosis in patients who have previously had Budd–Chiari syndrome, as they are at increased risk of rethrombosis.

Ultrasound features

- Expansion of vein: complete/partial loss of colour Doppler signal
- Internal echoes within vein
- Splenomegaly
- Ascites
- Colour Doppler:
  - intrahepatic collaterals
  - reversed/no flow in hepatic veins, possibly with stenotic segments
  - vein–vein shunting from one vein to another
- Spectral Doppler:
  - loss of normal hepatic vein triphasic waveform
  - waveform may be absent, turbulent, reversed or monophasic
  - reversed flow in IVC

What to look for

Scan image

4. Hepatic artery stenosis

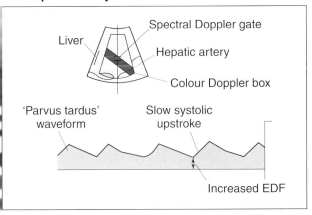

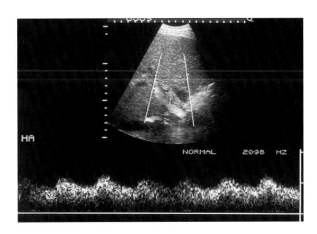

6a. Hepatic vein thrombosis colour Doppler

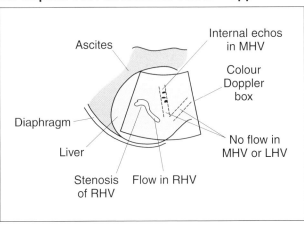

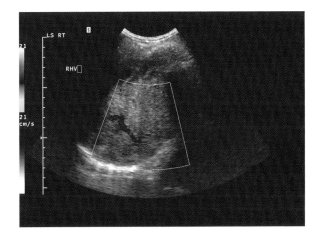

6b. Hepatic vein thrombosis spectral Doppler

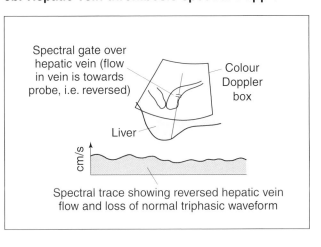

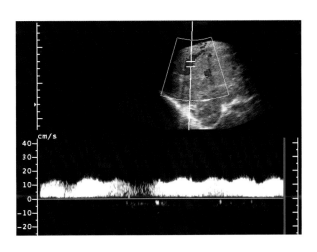

7

Testes

ANATOMY

(i) LS: anatomy

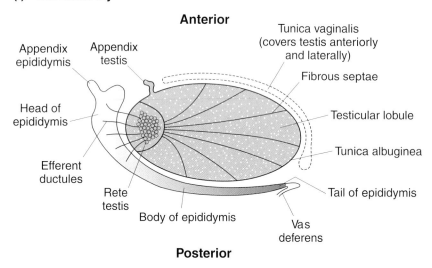

- Normal testis has a homogeneous echotexture.
- Fine echo-bright fibrous septae continuous with the tunica albuginea run through the gland, dividing it into lobules.
- Seminiferous tubules in the lobules converge to become larger straight tubules at the rete testis.
- The head of the epididymis contains converging tubules and is of a similar echotexture to the body of the testis.
- The body and tail of the epididymis appear more echo-poor.

(ii) TS: anatomy

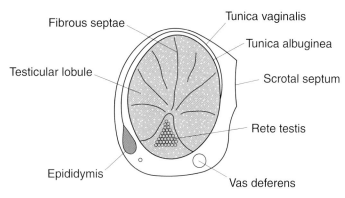

(iii) Arterial blood supply of testis

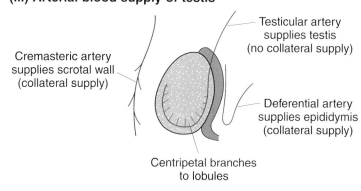

(iv) Venous drainage of testis

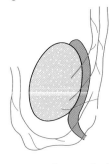

Venous drainage of right testis to inferior vena cava

Venous drainage of left testis to left renal vein

- The papiniform venous plexus drains the testis.
- The cremasteric plexus drains the epididymis and scrotal wall.
- Both freely anastamose.

PERFORMING THE SCAN

- **Preparation**: Obtain consent for the examination. A chaperone is advised for female examiners.
- **Patient position**: Supine with towel under scrotum. Ask the patient to hold the penis out of the way.
- **Probe**: High-frequency (6–10 MHz) linear.
- **Machine**: Select small-parts/testis preset mode, use multiple focal zones, turn off tissue harmonics, use parallel function and adjust the frequency to optimize images.
- **Method**: Acquire more than just representative images for each step if pathology is found.

Probe position	*Instructions*

1. LS: testis

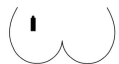

- Begin by placing the probe in the sagittal (LS) plane on the right testis.
- Look for the body of the testis and alter the depth until the epididymis can be seen behind it. Adjust the FOV accordingly.
- Scan through the testis in LS, observing:
  - normal homogeneous echotexture?
  - any masses, cysts or calcifications?
  - any peripheral fluid collections?
- Also observe the epididymis:
  - any swelling or echotexture abnormalities?
  - any cystic areas?
  - any dilated vessels posteriorly?
- Acquire a representative image.

2. TS: testis

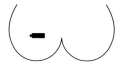

- Turn the probe 90° anticlockwise to scan in TS.
- Scan up and down through the testis and epididymis in this plane, observing for any pathology.
- Acquire a representative image.

What to look for

1.

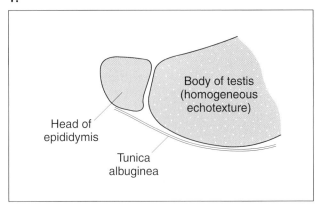

2.

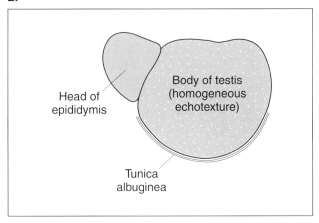

Scan image

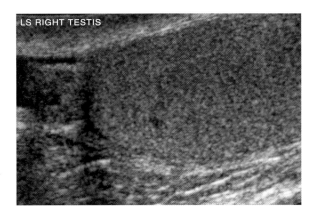

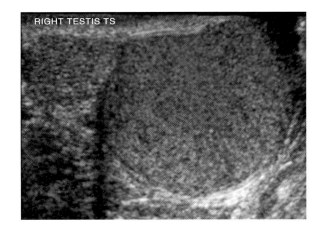

Probe position

3. **Testis lateral**

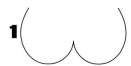

Instructions

- Place the probe on the lateral aspect of the right testis.
- Scan up and down through the gland in this plane, observing for any pathology as before.
- Acquire a representative image.

- Always remember to ask the patient which bit hurts or to show exactly where any lump is that they have felt.
- Make sure to scan carefully over this area.

Repeat all of the above on the left side.

Suspected varicocele

- Look for tortuous, dilated (>2 mm) veins posterior to the epididymis.
  Hint: 90% occur on the left side.
- Colour or power Doppler will demonstrate strong blood flow within them.
- Scanning as the patient strains or stands up should demonstrate that the vessels increase in size.
- Always perform a renal scan and renal vein Doppler after diagnosing a varicocele, as this can be associated with renal cell carcinoma.
- See the pathology section for more on this condition.

What to look for

3.

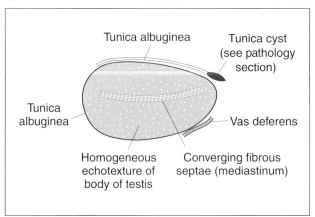

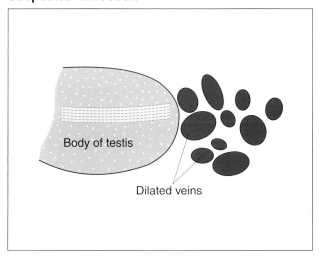

Suspected varicocele

Scan image

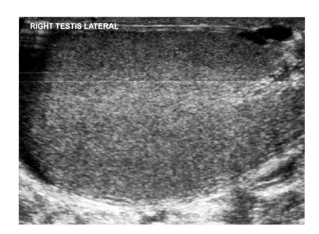

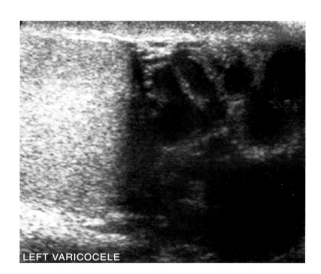

The painful testis (suspected torsion/epididymo-orchitis)

- Use power Doppler to evaluate blood flow in both testes.
- Optimize the Doppler signal: adjust the colour gain and focus position, magnify the image, reduce the colour box size, and set the filter and PRF at low.
- Look for normal perfusion, which should be out to the edges.
- If the painful testis has increased blood flow, this *may* be an orchitis.
- If the painful testis has reduced blood flow, this *may* be a torsion.
- See the pathology section for more on these conditions.

Infertility referral

- It is necessary to measure the testicular volumes (normal >10 cm^3).
- Calculate from LS and TS images, measuring the diameter in three planes.
- The split-screen function can be helpful for this.
- Use the measurement package to calculate the volume (on most machines).
- Remember to also examine carefully for secondary causes of subfertility, such as tumours and varicoceles.

Painful testis

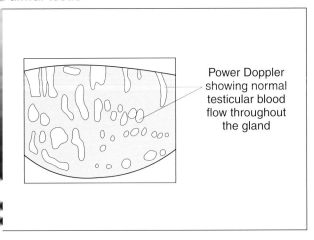

Power Doppler showing normal testicular blood flow throughout the gland

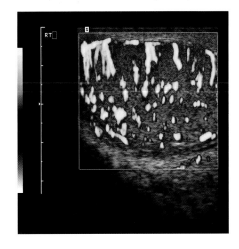

Infertility referral

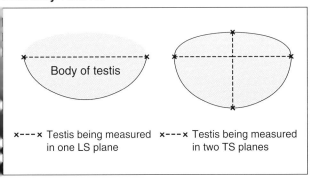

Body of testis

x---x Testis being measured in one LS plane x---x Testis being measured in two TS planes

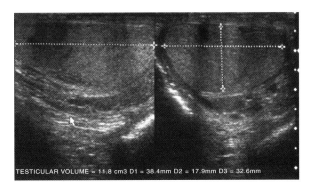

TESTICULAR VOLUME = 11.8 cm3 D1 = 38.4mm D2 = 17.9mm D3 = 32.6mm

TESTES: PATHOLOGY

1. Benign cystic lesions

(a) Intratesticular cyst

This is usually an incidental finding. Intratesticular cysts are located within the body of the testis and display typical features of a simple cyst:

- smooth edge
- thin wall
- echo-free contents
- postacoustic enhancement

(b) Epididymal cyst

This is a very common finding (up to 40% of men). It may present clinically as a smooth firm lump above the testis (caused by outpouchings of the epididymal tubules).

Ultrasound features
- Most commonly located in the epididymal head
- Displays the typical features of a simple cyst

(c) Tunica albuginea cyst

This presents clinically as a testicular lump, mimicking a tumour. This lesion is commonly discovered on self-examination, as it distorts the smooth testicular contour.

Ultrasound features
- Located on the periphery of the body of the testis (paratesticular)
- Displays the typical features of a simple cyst

What to look for

1a. Intratesticular cyst

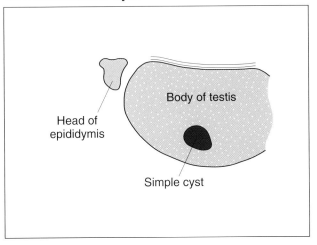

1b. Epididymal cyst

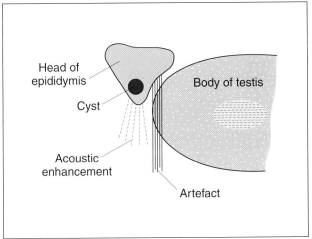

1c. Tunica albuginea cyst

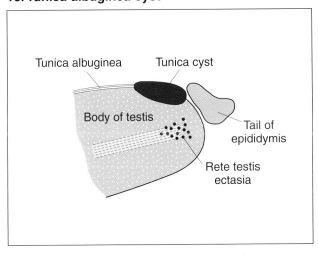

Scan image

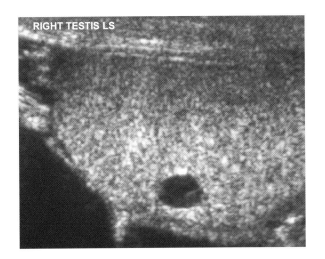

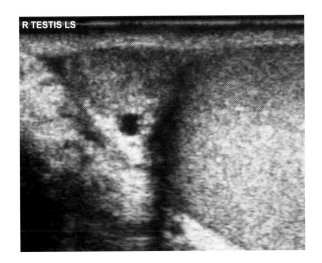

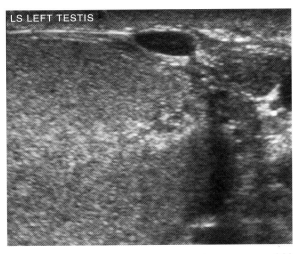

2. Hydrocele

This is fluid accumulation between the two layers of the tunica vaginalis. It can be congenital or acquired:

- Congenital: due to non-closure of the processus vaginalis
- Acquired: trauma, tumour, inflammation (these may contain debris)

Ultrasound features

- Seen as an echo-free area typically located on the anterolateral aspect of the testis
- Occasionally, fine septations or echo-bright debris may be seen within the fluid

3. Varicoceles

These are dilations of the papiniform veins that drain the testis, and are caused by incompetent vein valves. They are common (around 10% of males), with 90% occurring on the left side. Clinically, they may cause a dull scrotal ache and soft scrotal swelling.

Ultrasound features

- Seen as tortuous dilated (>2 mm) echo-free structures
- Located posterior to the epididymis
- The vessels increase in size on straining or standing upright
- The vessels show strong blood flow on colour or power Doppler

Rarely, a varicocele is due to a renal tumour obstructing venous return from the testicular veins. It is therefore important to always image the kidneys as well.

4. Postvasectomy changes

These are thought to be caused by a combination of back-pressure effects and low-grade inflammatory reaction. They are usually bilateral and asymptomatic.

Ultrasound features

- The epididymis appears thickened (>3 mm) and echo-poor, with multiple small punctate cystic areas

What to look for

2. Hydrocele

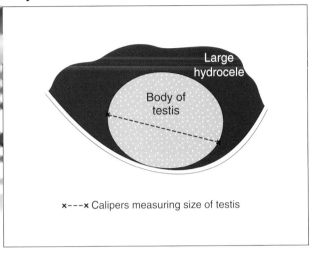

Large hydrocele

Body of testis

×---× Calipers measuring size of testis

3. Varicocele

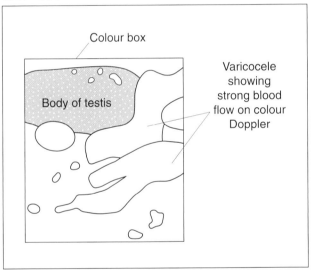

Colour box

Body of testis

Varicocele showing strong blood flow on colour Doppler

4. Postvasectomy change

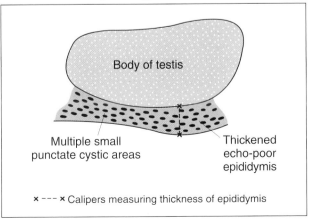

Body of testis

Multiple small punctate cystic areas

Thickened echo-poor epididymis

×---× Calipers measuring thickness of epididymis

Scan image

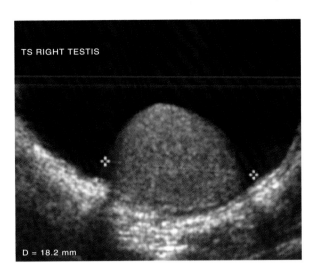

TS RIGHT TESTIS

D = 18.2 mm

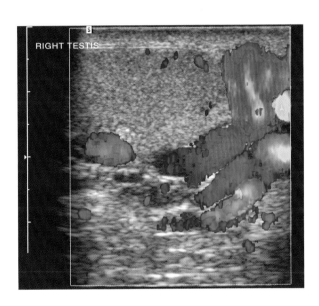

RIGHT TESTIS

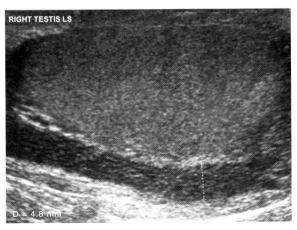

RIGHT TESTIS LS

D = 4.8 mm

143

5. Testicular microlithiasis

These multiple small calcific foci are usually an incidental finding, but some studies have shown an increased risk of developing a testicular malignancy. They are also associated with subfertility.

Ultrasound features

• More than 5 echo-bright foci (each <3 mm) within the body of the testis

Follow-up protocol as per Leeds Teaching Hospitals

• Age <40 years: annual ultrasound advised
• Age >40 years: no routine ultrasound follow-up

(in both groups regular self-examination is recommended)

Hint: These are not to be confused with larger solitary areas of calcification that can be seen within testicular tumours and in some postinflammatory conditions.

6. Testicular tumours

As a rule, most intratesticular mass lesions are malignant. The most common tumour type is the seminoma.

Ultrasound features

• Variable appearances: tumours can appear as echo-poor, cystic or mixed echogenicity mass lesions

Note: Remember to do an abdominal/pelvic scan and request a chest X-ray to assess for secondary disease. A urologist should be contacted immediately with the result (even if the patient is a GP referral).

What to look for

5. Testicular microlithiasis

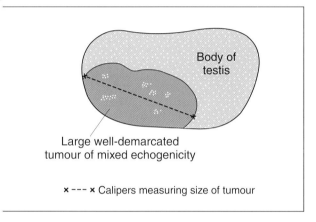

Body of testis

Microcalcifications

6a. Testicular tumour

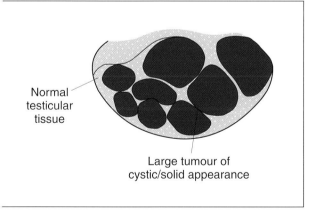

Large well-demarcated
tumour of mixed echogenicity

Body of
testis

✕ --- ✕ Calipers measuring size of tumour

6b. Testicular tumour

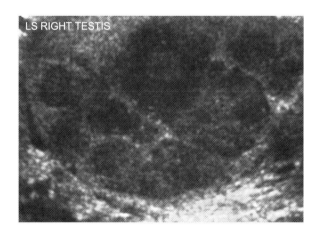

Normal
testicular
tissue

Large tumour of
cystic/solid appearance

Scan image

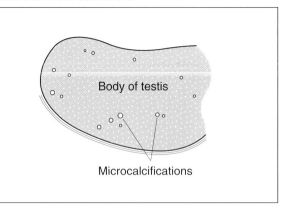

LS RIGHT TESTIS

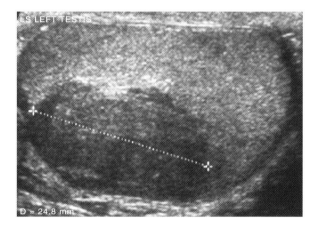

LS LEFT TESTIS

D = 24.8 mm

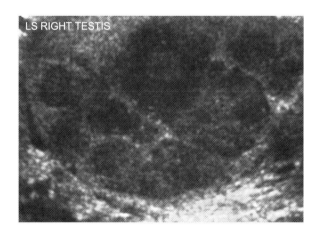

LS RIGHT TESTIS

7. Epididymo-orchitis

This is caused by ascending spread of infection (e.g. chlamydia, gonorrhoea) or by the blood-borne route (e.g. mumps). It is commonly seen in young males. The majority of cases are unilateral and of epididymitis only.

Ultrasound features

- Epididymis appears swollen (>3 mm) and of mixed echogenicity; the tail is the most common part affected
- Colour/power Doppler flow is increased over the affected area in the acute phase
- There may be a reactive hydrocele
- Oedematous thickening of overlying scrotal skin is common
- Rarely, the condition can progress to abscess formation
- If the testis is involved, this appears swollen, with echo-poor areas (uniform or focal)
- Colour/power Doppler flow in the testes is increased, but in very severe cases it may be reduced, causing diagnostic confusion with testicular torsion

8. Testicular torsion

This is twisting of the spermatic cord resulting in testicular ischaemia. It is usually caused by the 'bell-clapper' anatomical variant, in which the tunica vaginalis extends around posterior to the testis, allowing it to twist more easily. Torsion can be complete (360° twist), partial or intermittent (torsion/detorsion).

Ultrasound features

- Testis appears echo-poor; it often has a reactive hydrocele
- The hallmark is reduced/absent intratesticular blood flow using power Doppler (see earlier). Note that the epididymis may show increased flow, as it has a collateral blood supply

Note:
- Beware false-positives: severe epididymo-orchitis
- Beware false-negatives: intermittent torsion/detorsion

This is an emergency, and if there is strong clinical suspicion, taking the patient straight to theatre should not be delayed.

What to look for

7. Epididymo-orchitis

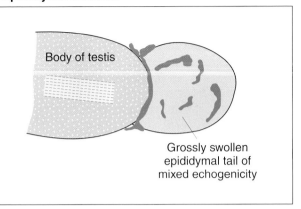

Body of testis

Grossly swollen epididymal tail of mixed echogenicity

8a. Testicular torsion

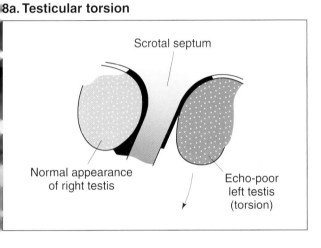

Scrotal septum

Normal appearance of right testis

Echo-poor left testis (torsion)

8b. Testicular torsion

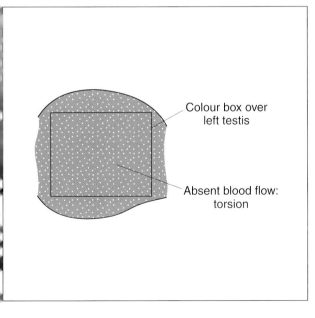

Colour box over left testis

Absent blood flow: torsion

Scan image

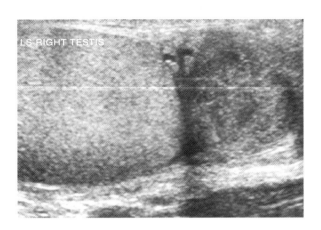

LS RIGHT TESTIS

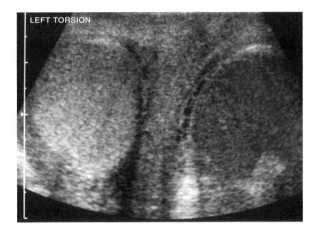

LEFT TORSION

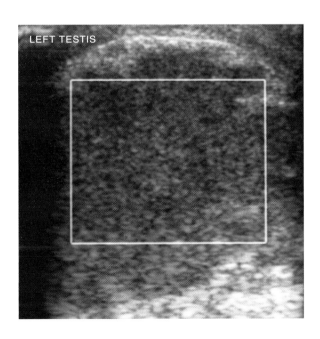

LEFT TESTIS

9. Torsion of testicular appendix

Presents with sudden-onset of scrotal pain and swelling; this can mimic testicular torsion. However, the condition requires no surgical intervention and resolves spontaneously. The appendix will often detach itself and come to lie free within the scrotal sac, where it may calcify to become a scrotolith (scrotal pearl).

Ultrasound features

• Acutely, the appendix appears enlarged due to oedema, often with a reactive hydrocele

• A scrotolith is a small mobile echo-bright structure within the scrotal sac

What to look for

9. Torsion of testicular appendix

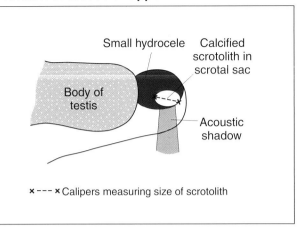

Small hydrocele   Calcified
scrotolith in
scrotal sac

Body of
testis

Acoustic
shadow

✗ – – – ✗ Calipers measuring size of scrotolith

Scan image

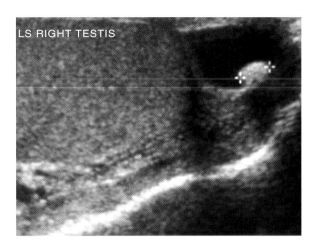

LS RIGHT TESTIS

8

Lower limb veins

ANATOMY

Deep veins of right leg

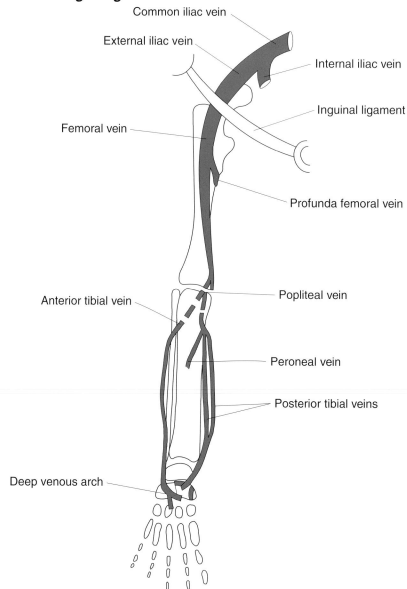

Common iliac vein

External iliac vein

Internal iliac vein

Inguinal ligament

Femoral vein

Profunda femoral vein

Popliteal vein

Anterior tibial vein

Peroneal vein

Posterior tibial veins

Deep venous arch

Superficial veins of right leg

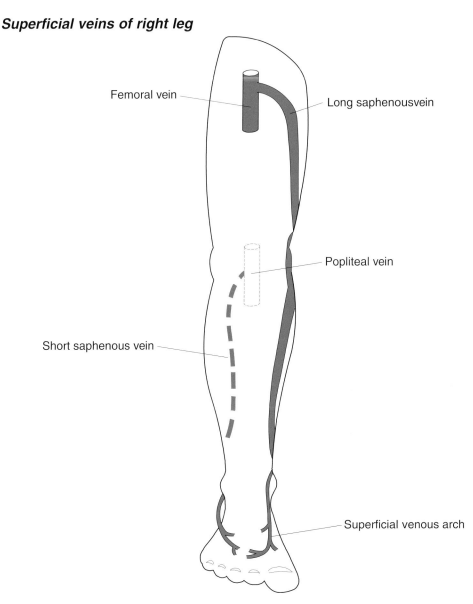

Femoral vein

Long saphenousvein

Popliteal vein

Short saphenous vein

Superficial venous arch

Key points

1. The superficial veins drain into the deep veins.
2. The deep veins and perforating veins contain valves.
3. 25% of people have duplicated femoral or popliteal veins – always scan both vessel lumens (3% have triple femoral or popliteal veins).
4. The femoral vein is *deep* to the femoral artery.
5. The popliteal vein is *superficial* to the popliteal artery.

PERFORMING THE SCAN

- **Patient position**: Sit up with leg exposed from groin to toes.
- **Preparation**: Nil.
- **Probe**: High-frequency (5–8 MHz) linear (for a very obese/swollen leg, consider using a low-frequency (3–5 MHz) curvilinear probe).
- **Machine**: Select the venous vascular preset mode. Use tissue harmonics if the SNR is poor. Use a dual screen when acquiring images with and without compression in TS.
- **Method**: Start at the groin and scan distally. If a thrombus is found:
  (a) STOP scanning distally, as there is a risk of dislodging the thrombus.
  (b) Scan proximally to examine the extent of the thrombus, i.e. if there is femoral vein DVT, scan the iliac vein; if there is iliac vein DVT, scan the IVC, etc.
  (c) Use colour flow to distinguish occlusive versus non-occlusive thrombus.

Always scan the bit that the patient says hurts.

Probe position	*Instructions*
1. TS: proximal femoral vein 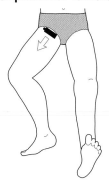	• Sit patient up to increase venous congestion. The patient bends the knee and externally rotates the hip so that the leg falls out laterally. • Place the probe in the groin crease to find the proximal femoral vein in TS. Adjust the focus to the level of the vessel. • Look for the 'Mickey Mouse sign' – the head of Mickey is the femoral vein, and the ears are the femoral artery (laterally) and the long saphenous vein (medially). • Compress the vein with the probe: – complete compression of the vein = no thrombus – partial or no compression = thrombus • Acquire one image without compression and one image with compression.
2. TS: mid femoral vein 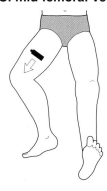	• Keep scanning in TS. • Follow the femoral vein down to mid-thigh. • Compress intermittently, i.e. every 1 cm: – complete compression of the vein = no thrombus – partial or no compression = thrombus • Increase the depth on descending the leg. • Keep the focus at the level of the vessel. • Use colour Doppler to aid in locating the vein. • Acquire one image without compression and one image with compression.

What to look for

1. (Dual screen)

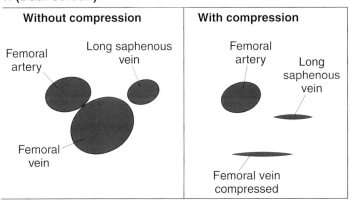

Without compression	With compression
Femoral artery	Femoral artery
Long saphenous vein	Long saphenous vein
Femoral vein	Femoral vein compressed

2.

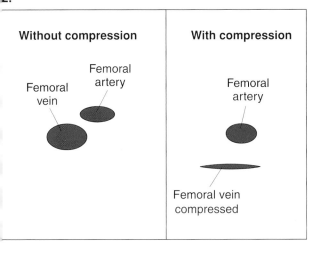

Without compression	With compression
Femoral vein	Femoral artery
Femoral artery	Femoral vein compressed

Scan image

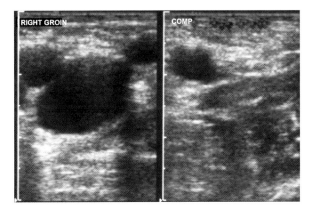

RIGHT GROIN   COMP

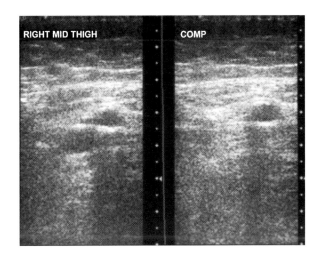

RIGHT MID THIGH   COMP

Probe position	*Instructions*

3. TS: distal femoral vein

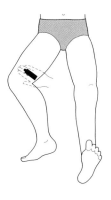

- Keep scanning in TS.
- Follow the course of the femoral vein down to the knee, and continue to compress intermittently.
- At the lower one-third of the thigh, the femoral vein enters the adductor canal, and it becomes more difficult to compress the vein against the femur. Therefore, try putting the free hand under the leg and pushing up against the probe to test for full compression.
- Acquire one image without compression and one image with compression.

4. LS: femoral vein

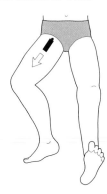

- Now scan the femoral vein in LS.
- Go back to the groin and find the femoral vein first in TS; then rotate the probe through 90° clockwise to scan in LS.
- Follow the femoral vein down to the knee. Look for small non-occlusive thrombi in the vessel wall, especially around the valves.
- Turn on colour Doppler and set the PRF, colour gain and wall filter etc. to optimize edge definition and avoid colour flow bleeding out of the vein.
- Scan the femoral vein again in LS with colour, looking for filling defects, i.e. non-occlusive thrombi. Measure any abnormalities seen (size of thrombus, lymph nodes, etc.).
- Acquire one or two representative images.

5. TS: popliteal vein

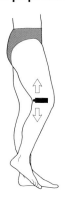

- Now scan the popliteal vein in TS.
- Ask the patient to roll away onto the left side and to slightly flex the knee.
- Place the probe in the popliteal fossa and look for the popliteal vein (more superficial than the artery).
- Push with the probe against the posterior tibia to check for complete compression. (If this method proves difficult to use, see the appendix to this protocol for alternative methods.)
- Acquire one image without compression and one image with compression.

What to look for   ## *Scan image*

3. (Dual screen)

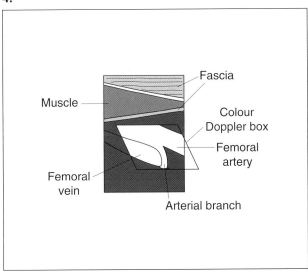

Without compression	With compression
Duplicated femoral veins	Compressed femoral veins
Femoral artery	Femoral artery

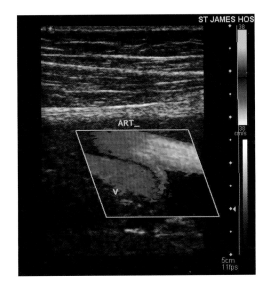

4.

Fascia

Muscle

Colour Doppler box

Femoral artery

Femoral vein

Arterial branch

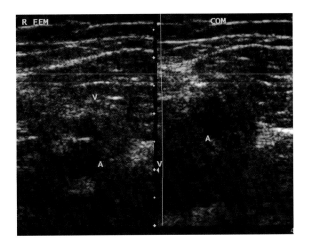

5. (Dual screen)

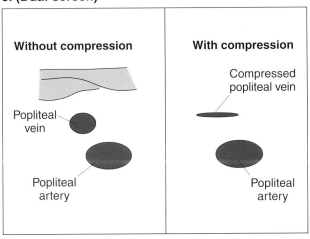

Without compression	With compression
Popliteal vein	Compressed popliteal vein
Popliteal artery	Popliteal artery

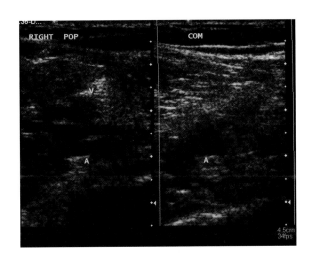

Probe position

6. LS: popliteal vein

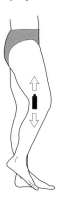

Instructions

- Now scan the popliteal vein(s) in LS. To do this, find the popliteal vein in TS and then rotate the probe through 90° clockwise.
- Look for small non-occlusive thrombi on the vessel wall.
- Turn on colour Doppler and scan the popliteal vein again in LS, looking for filling defects, i.e. non-occlusive thrombi.
- Measure any abnormalities seen.
- Acquire representative image(s).

7. LS: posterior tibial veins

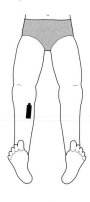

- Now scan the posterior tibial veins.
- Ask the patient to sit up again and place the probe medial to the tibial spine.
- Look for three calf vessels: two posterior tibial veins laterally and one posterior tibial artery in between. It is easiest to start mid-tibia and then scan up and down the vessels. The veins are often difficult to visualize without colour Doppler.
- Put colour on (there is usually very little flow). To check for patency, squeeze the ankle and look for increased flow in the veins.
- Acquire one image without ankle squeezing and one image with squeezing.

What to look for   **Scan image**

6.

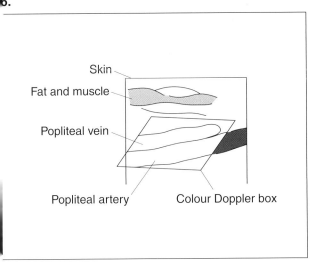

Skin

Fat and muscle

Popliteal vein

Popliteal artery   Colour Doppler box

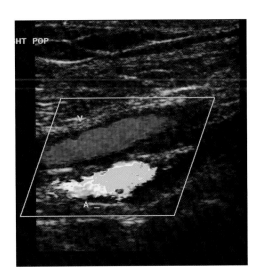

7.

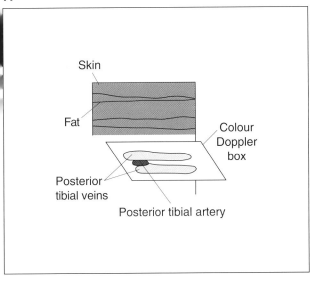

Skin

Fat

Colour Doppler box

Posterior tibial veins

Posterior tibial artery

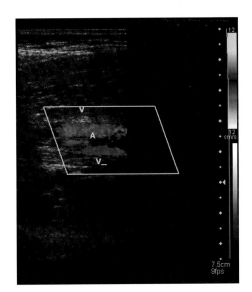

Appendix to Step 5: Alternative techniques to scan the popliteal vessels

There are three commonly used techniques to scan the popliteal vessels. The ideal technique largely depends on the patient, and technique must be adapted depending on their age, comorbidity and degree of immobility.

Patient position	Advantages	Disadvantages
1. Posterior oblique; knee flexed 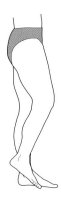	• This position is well-tolerated by the patient • Probe access is easy • It is easy to compress the vein	• It is difficult to achieve this position in patients with OA or fracture of the pelvis/hip
2. Prone; knee slightly flexed 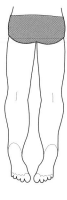	• Probe access is easy • It is easy to compress the vein in a young patient	• Elderly patients' veins compress/collapse with no/little pressure • This is a difficult position for some patients to achieve

Patient position

3. Sitting with foot flat on couch and knee flexed to 90°

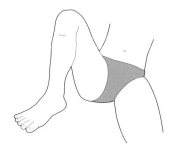

Advantages

- This is a good position for immobile patients

Disadvantages

- It is a difficult position for patients with painful/swollen legs
- Excess pressure is required to compress the vein due to venous congestion
- Probe access is difficult

LOWER LIMBS: COMMON PATHOLOGY

1. Deep vein thrombosis

Risk factors include age, immobility, IVDU, malignancy, obesity, OCP, pregnancy and surgery. DVT presents as a painful swollen limb. The differential diagnosis includes cellulitis, ruptured Baker's cyst and haematoma.

The scan should be repeated after 1 week if symptoms/signs of a thrombosis persist despite a normal scan.

Ultrasound features
- Acute (<1 week): echo-free thrombus in a swollen vein
- Chronic: echo-bright thrombus in a contracted vein, sometimes with tortuous recanalization

	Occlusion due to thrombosis	*Stenosis due to thrombosis*
TS with compression	Non-compressible	Incompletely compressible
LS with colour Doppler	No flow	Filling defect
LS with spectral Doppler	No flow	Increased velocity at stenosis

What to look for

1a. DVT in TS (Dual screen)

Without compression

Femoral
artery

Femoral
vein

With compression

Femoral
artery

Femoral vein
not completely
compressible

1b. DVT in LS

Skin

Fat

Vein

Thrombus

1c. DVT with colour Doppler

Thrombus
in popliteal
vein

Colour Doppler box

No blood flow

Popliteal artery
with blood flow
demonstrated

Scan image

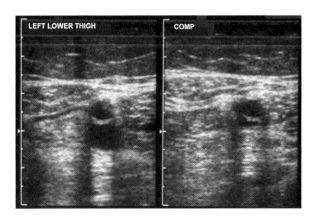

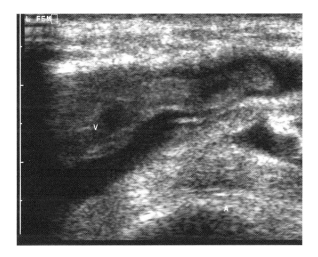

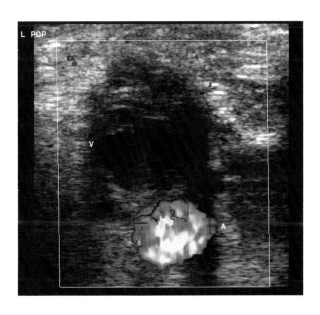

2. Baker's cyst

Baker's cysts arise between the medial head of the gastrocnemius and the semimembranosus tendons. They cause pain and swelling when they rupture.

Ultrasound features

- Found on medial side of the popliteal fossa
- Oval/crescent shape
- Usually echo-free
- Communicates with the knee joint
- When the cyst ruptures, it may extend into the calf, causing swelling

3. Haematoma

This can mimic a DVT (i.e. pain and limb swelling). It is usually due to a muscle tear or external trauma.

Ultrasound features

- Within soft tissues/muscles
- Well-defined margins
- Predominantly echo-poor; may contain echo-bright fibrin strands

4. Cellulitis

This is infection of the subcutaneous tissues. It presents with a hot, painful, swollen and red limb (or any affected area of the body).

Ultrasound features

- Oedema: fluid between subcutaneous fat, resulting in a 'crazy-paving' effect
- Hyperaemic flow in the vessels

What to look for

2. Baker's cyst

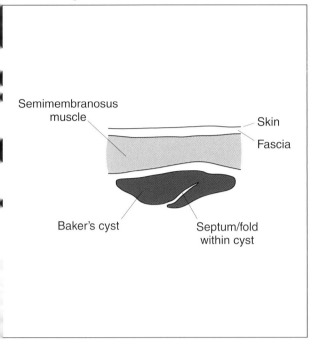

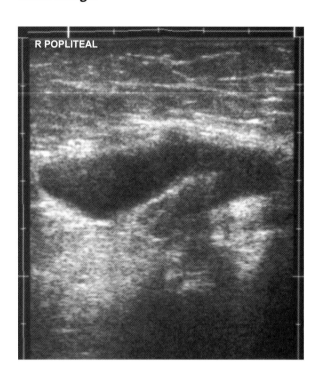

3. Haematoma

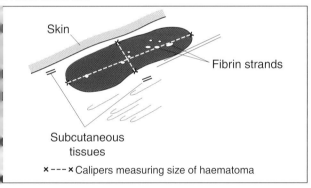

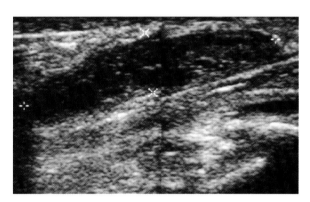

4. Cellulitis

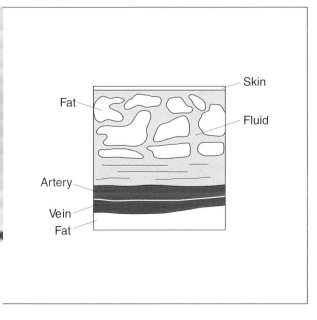

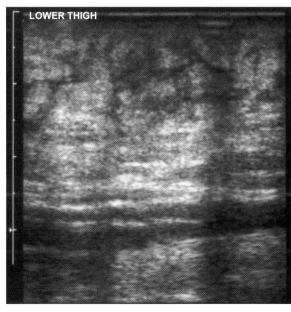

5. Thrombophlebitis

This is inflammation, possibly with thrombosis, of the superficial veins, e.g. LSV and SSV.

Ultrasound features
- Superficial vessel wall is irregular/ragged
- Vessel is still compressible

Hint: Check that the thrombus does not extend to the deep system veins.

6. Varicose veins

These are dilated tortuous superficial veins. Risk factors include age, pregnancy, family history and obesity.

Ultrasound features
- Dilated tortuous superficial veins

7. Lymphadenopathy

Common causes include infection (local or systemic), metastases and lymphoma. It may increase suspicion of cellulitis versus DVT (but keep in mind that the two can coexist!).

Ultrasound features of a normal lymph node
- Elliptical
- Long axis <10 mm, short axis <7 mm
- Echo-bright hilum of fat
- Echo-poor cortex

Ultrasound features of an abnormal lymph node
- Spherical
- Long axis >10 mm
- Loss of echo-bright hilum
- May exert mass effect on surrounding structures

What to look for

5. Thrombophlebitis

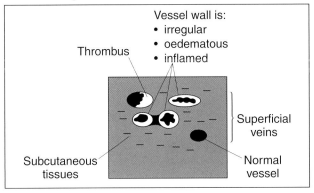

Vessel wall is:
- irregular
- oedematous
- inflamed

Thrombus

Superficial veins

Subcutaneous tissues

Normal vessel

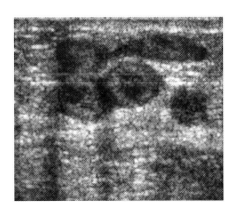

6. Varicose vein

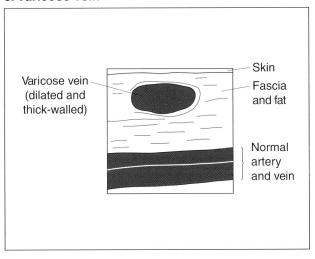

Varicose vein (dilated and thick-walled)

Skin

Fascia and fat

Normal artery and vein

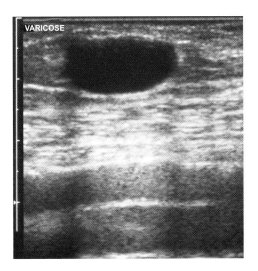

VARICOSE

7. Lymph node

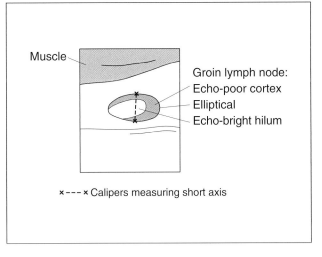

Muscle

Groin lymph node:
Echo-poor cortex
Elliptical
Echo-bright hilum

×---× Calipers measuring short axis

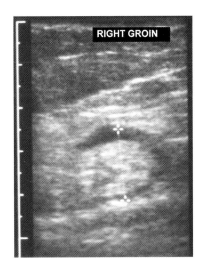

RIGHT GROIN

9

Carotid Doppler examination

ANATOMY

The great vessels

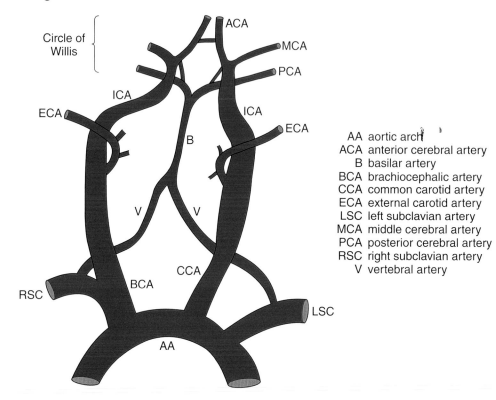

AA aortic arch
ACA anterior cerebral artery
B basilar artery
BCA brachiocephalic artery
CCA common carotid artery
ECA external carotid artery
LSC left subclavian artery
MCA middle cerebral artery
PCA posterior cerebral artery
RSC right subclavian artery
V vertebral artery

Key points

1. The ICA has no branches extracranially.
2. One vertebral artery tends to be more dominant than the other: usually left > right.
3. If the CCA is occluded, there are two collateral pathways, via:
    (i) the circle of Willis
    (ii) the ophthalmic artery

PERFORMING THE SCAN

- **Patient position**: Neck extended with head turned to contralateral side.
- **Preparation**: Nil.
- **Probe**: High-frequency (7.5 MHz) linear.
- **Machine**: Select arterial vascular preset mode. Use tissue harmonics if the SNR is poor. Set the focus to the posterior wall of the vessel.
- **Method**: Do not apply any pressure with the probe. Start at the root of the neck and scan cranially along the course of the vessels. Scan both sides of the neck.

Probe position

1. TS: common carotid artery

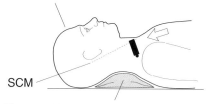

Neck extended and head turned to contralateral side

SCM

Place a pillow under the patient's neck to achieve optimal position

Instructions

- Begin by placing the probe in TS over the root of the neck, i.e. at the CCA origin.
- Use the SCM as a window to scan through. If the vessel image is not clear, try scanning anterior or posterior to the SCM instead.
- Follow the course of the carotid arteries up the neck as high as possible.
- Look for:
  - level of CCA bifurcation
  - evidence of arterial disease
- Measure any abnormalities seen.
- Acquire representative image(s).

2. LS: carotid arteries

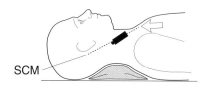

SCM

- Now scan the carotid arteries in LS. To do this, first scan the CCA origin in TS as in Step 1 and then rotate the probe through 90° clockwise so that the CCA is now imaged in LS.
- Follow the course of the carotid arteries up the neck as high as possible.
- The ICA and ECA are in different planes: therefore find the CCA bifurcation, keep the lower portion of the probe over the CCA, and rotate the upper portion through small angles to image the ICA then the ECA separately.
- Look for:
  - atheromatous plaques
  - intima–media thickening (below the CCA bulb, it should be <0.8 mm).
- Acquire representative image(s).

What to look for

Scan image

1.

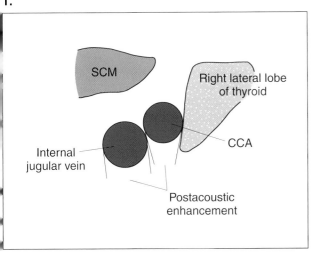

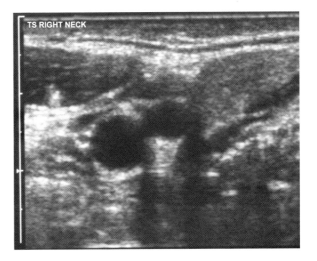

2.

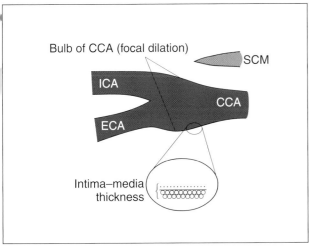

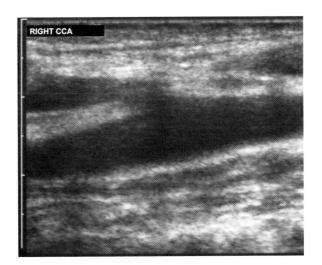

Probe position	**Instructions**

3. LS: colour Doppler carotid arteries

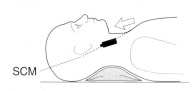

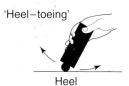
SCM

'Heel–toeing'

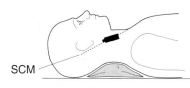
Heel · Toe

- Keep scanning the carotids in LS. Turn on colour Doppler and place the colour box over the vessel. Steer the box so that the angle of the box is in the same direction as the vessel flow. 'Heel–toeing' the probe may help get a good angle of Doppler resonation.
- Optimize the colour signal: adjust the colour gain and focus position, narrow the FOV and reduce the colour box size. Set the PRF so that colour aliasing occurs mid-vessel during peak-systole.
- Follow the course of the CCA, ICA and ECA up the neck in LS.
- Look for:
  - small branches to identify the ECA
  - velocity change/colour aliasing (stenosis)
  - filling defects (atheromatous plaques)
  - absence of flow (occlusion)
- Acquire representative image(s).

4. LS: spectral Doppler CCA

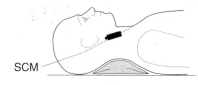
SCM

- Keep scanning in LS with colour Doppler. Select a segment of the CCA. If a stenosis has already been demonstrated, select this segment.
- Now turn on spectral Doppler and place the gate over the CCA at the point of maximum peak velocity, acquiring a trace. Optimize the waveform by adjusting the gate size and ensuring a beam-flow angle of 0°–60°.
- Select 'calculations' on the machine and then measure the peak velocity. (If no flow is detected with colour Doppler, increase the colour gain and reduce the PRF to increase the sensitivity. If there is still no flow detected, the vessel is occluded.)
- Acquire one or two spectral waveforms.
  Hint: Remember to steer the colour box so that its angle is in the same direction as the vessel flow.

5. LS: spectral Doppler ECA

SCM

- Repeat Step 4 for the ECA.
- The normal ECA waveform is:
  - pulsatile with a characteristic notch
  - high resistance flow
  - low diastolic flow
- Acquire one or two spectral waveforms.

Hint

It can sometimes be difficult to identify the ECA versus the ICA. Remember that the ECA:

- has extracranial branches – use colour Doppler to help identify them
- demonstrates the 'temporal tapping' phenomena – tap the temporal artery in front of the ear and look for alteration in the spectral waveform of the ECA (there is no effect on the ICA waveform)

What to look for

Scan image

3.

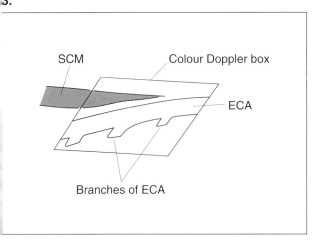

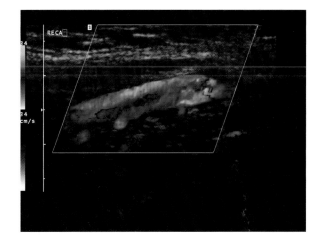

4.

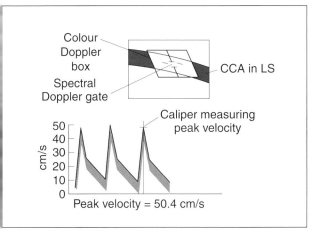

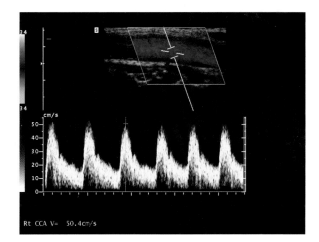

5.

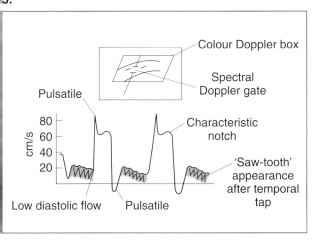

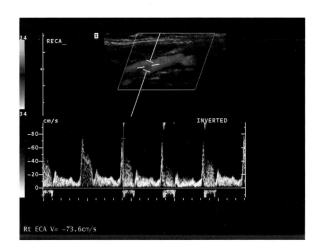

Probe position	**Instructions**

6. LS: spectral Doppler ICA

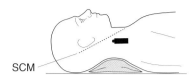

SCM

- Repeat Step 4 for the ICA.
- Measure peak velocity.
- The normal ICA waveform is:
  - less pulsatile than the ECA
  - low resistance flow
  - higher diastolic flow
- Acquire one or two spectral waveforms.

Hint: Ensure the beam to flow angle is 0°–60° for accurate velocity measurements.

7. LS: colour Doppler vertebral artery

Angle probe towards C-spine

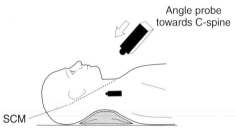

SCM

- Now scan the vertebral artery in LS. Turn off spectral Doppler and keep only colour Doppler switched on.
- To locate the vertebral artery:
  - First find the mid CCA in LS
  - Then angle the probe posteriorly in the direction of the cervical spine
  - Increase the depth and deepen the focus position
  - Look for the vertebral processes (bright echoes) – the vertebral artery and vein lie between them and appear as 'flashes' of colour
- Acquire a representative image.

8. LS: spectral Doppler vertebral artery

Angle probe towards C-spine

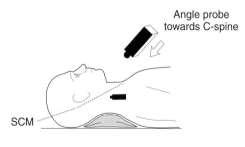

SCM

- Now turn on spectral Doppler and place the gate over the vessel to acquire a spectral waveform as described in Step 4.
- Record the direction of flow only.
- Acquire one or two spectral waveforms.

9. Contralateral-side neck vessels

- Repeat Steps 1–7 for the vessels on the opposite side of the neck.

Hint: Do not stand the patient up straight away at the end of the examination, as they are at risk of a vasovagal episode.

What to look for

Scan image

6.

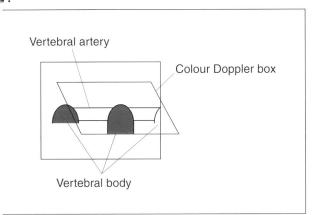

Spectral Doppler gate

ICA

Caliper measuring peak velocity (~100 cm/s)

Colour Doppler box over ICA

High EDF, i.e. blood flows always toward the brain (~50 cm/s = normal)

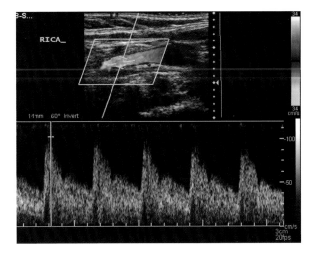

7.

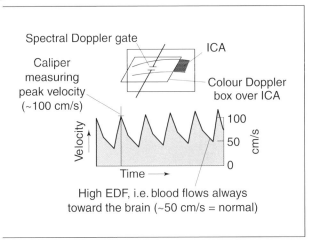

Vertebral artery

Colour Doppler box

Vertebral body

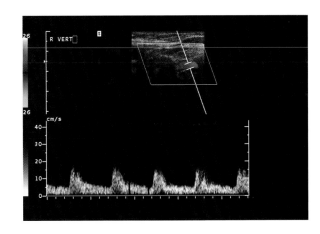

8.

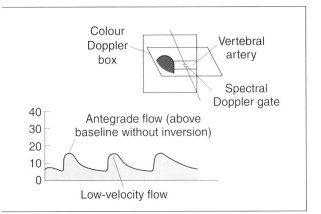

Colour Doppler box

Vertebral artery

Spectral Doppler gate

Antegrade flow (above baseline without inversion)

Low-velocity flow

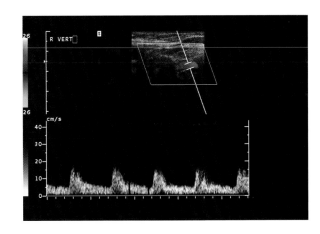

PATHOLOGY

1. Atheromatous plaques

Atherosclerosis is a disease of large and medium-sized muscular arteries. It is characterized by the accumulation of lipids, calcium and cellular debris within the intima of the vessel wall, forming atheromatous plaques. These plaques result in luminal obstruction, abnormalities of blood flow, and diminished oxygen supply to target organs. The major risk factors are smoking, hypercholesterolaemia, diabetes and hypertension.

Ultrasound features
- Localized irregular thickening of the vessel wall (measure in TS and LS) causing stenosis
- The echogenicity of the plaque depends on its contents:
  - echo-poor: blood- or lipid-filled = increased risk of rupture
  - echo-bright: calcified = more benign
- With colour Doppler:
  - filling defect
  - aliasing
  - no flow (complete occlusion)
- With spectral Doppler:
  - increased peak velocity
  - spectral broadening

There are five types of atheromatous plaques, graded according to their ultrasound appearance:

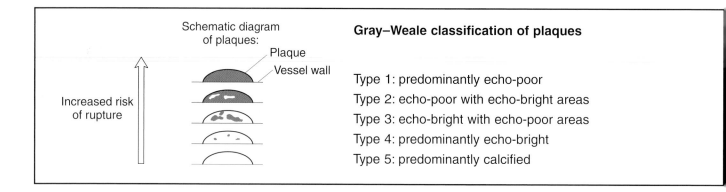

Gray–Weale classification of plaques

Type 1: predominantly echo-poor
Type 2: echo-poor with echo-bright areas
Type 3: echo-bright with echo-poor areas
Type 4: predominantly echo-bright
Type 5: predominantly calcified

Across a stenosis:
- The peak velocity of the blood increases in proportion to the degree of stenosis.
- The normal characteristic waveform of the vessel is altered.
- There is spectral broadening of the waveform, representing turbulent blood flow.

Therefore, by using spectral Doppler to measure the peak velocity, the degree of stenosis can be estimated. There are many different peak-systolic velocity cut-off values to determine ICA stenosis. As an example the following values are used in Leeds Teaching Hospitals (see Table below). However it is recommended that the agreed cut-off values in your radiology department are used as there is considerable variation between hospitals.

Peak-systolic velocity (m/s)	Degree of stenosis (%)	Management
<1.5	0–49	Medical
1.5–2.3	50–69	Medical
>2.3	>70	Surgical
None	Occluded	Medical

What to look for

1a. Intimal thickening

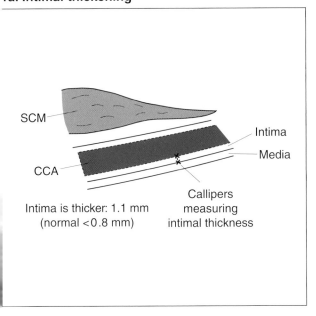

SCM

CCA

Intima

Media

Callipers measuring intimal thickness

Intima is thicker: 1.1 mm
(normal <0.8 mm)

1b. Echo-bright plaque

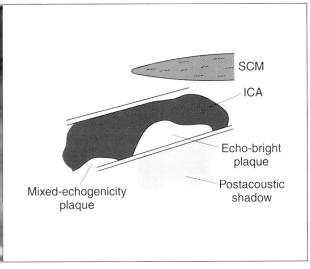

SCM

ICA

Echo-bright plaque

Postacoustic shadow

Mixed-echogenicity plaque

1c. Echo-poor plaque

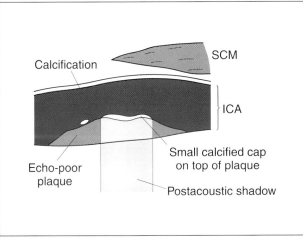

Calcification

SCM

ICA

Echo-poor plaque

Small calcified cap on top of plaque

Postacoustic shadow

1d, e, f overleaf

Scan image

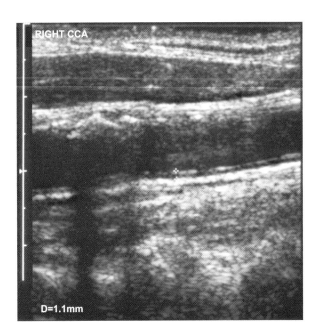

RIGHT CCA

D=1.1mm

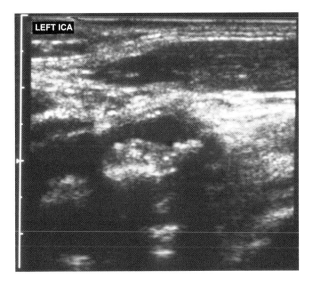

LEFT ICA

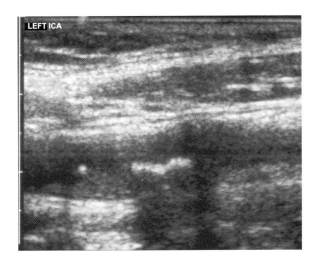

LEFT ICA

What to look for

1d. Spectral Doppler 0–49% ICA stenosis

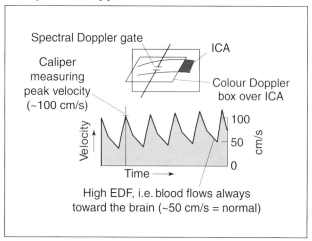

Spectral Doppler gate

ICA

Caliper measuring peak velocity (~100 cm/s)

Colour Doppler box over ICA

Velocity

Time →

100
50
0
cm/s

High EDF, i.e. blood flows always toward the brain (~50 cm/s = normal)

1e. Spectral Doppler 50–69% ICA stenosis

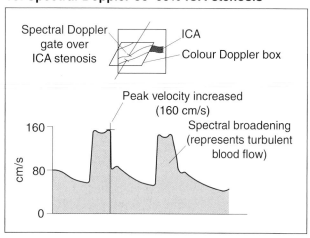

Spectral Doppler gate over ICA stenosis

ICA

Colour Doppler box

Peak velocity increased (160 cm/s)

Spectral broadening (represents turbulent blood flow)

160
80
0
cm/s

1f. Spectral Doppler >70% ICA stenosis

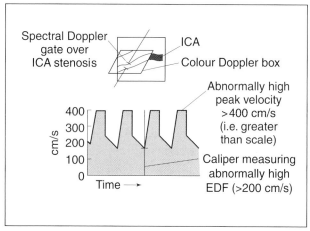

Spectral Doppler gate over ICA stenosis

ICA

Colour Doppler box

Abnormally high peak velocity >400 cm/s (i.e. greater than scale)

Caliper measuring abnormally high EDF (>200 cm/s)

400
300
200
100
0
cm/s

Time →

Scan image

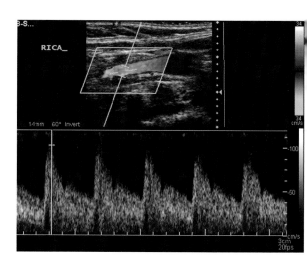

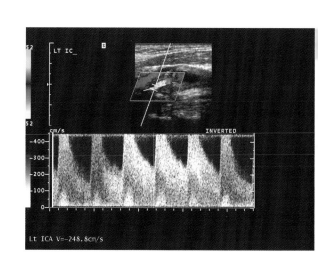

2. Subclavian steal syndrome

This is due to occlusion of the proximal subclavian (or brachiocephalic) artery – i.e. it is usually due to an occlusive atheromatous plaque. Blood flows in a *retrograde* direction down the same-side vertebral artery to supply the distal subclavian artery.

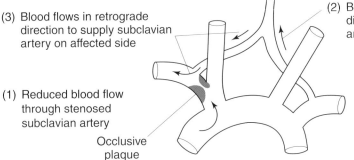

(3) Blood flows in retrograde direction to supply subclavian artery on affected side

(2) Blood flows in antegrade direction up vertebral artery on unaffected side

(1) Reduced blood flow through stenosed subclavian artery

Occlusive plaque

Ultrasound features

- Plaque seen in subclavian (or brachiocephalic) artery
- Absence of flow in subclavian (or brachiocephalic) artery with colour Doppler
- Retrograde flow in unilateral vertebral artery

What to look for

2a. Normal vertebral spectral Doppler

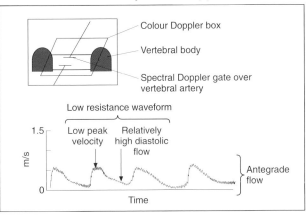

Colour Doppler box

Vertebral body

Spectral Doppler gate over vertebral artery

Low resistance waveform

Low peak velocity

Relatively high diastolic flow

Antegrade flow

Time

2b. Partial subclavian steal spectral Doppler

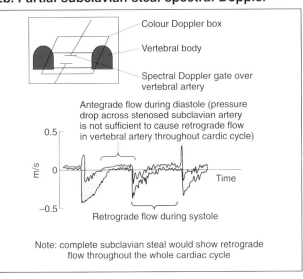

Colour Doppler box

Vertebral body

Spectral Doppler gate over vertebral artery

Antegrade flow during diastole (pressure drop across stenosed subclavian artery is not sufficient to cause retrograde flow in vertebral artery throughout cardic cycle)

Retrograde flow during systole

Note: complete subclavian steal would show retrograde flow throughout the whole cardiac cycle

Scan image

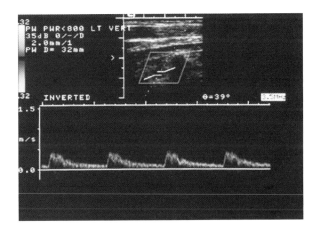

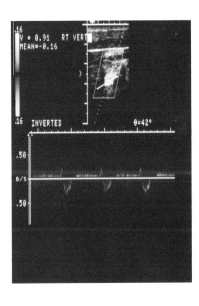

10
Female pelvis

ANATOMY

(i) LS: anatomy

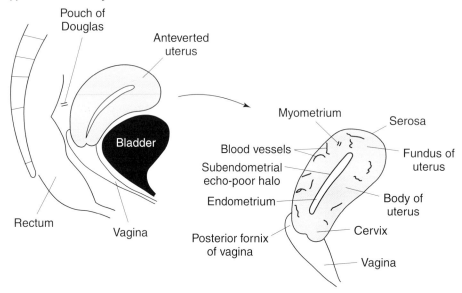

- 80% of women will have an anteverted or anteflexed uterus.
- Normal myometrium is of a homogenous echotexture. Fine echo-poor vessels can be seen within it.
- Endometrium is echo-bright (appearances vary with menstrual cycle – see (iv)).
- Endometrium is surrounded by an echo-poor subendometrial halo, which represents a rim of compacted myometrium.
- It is normal to see a trace of free fluid in the Pouch of Douglas postovulation.
- Note that LS and TS ultrasound planes in the pelvis are defined in relation to the uterus, which often lies deviated to one side.

(ii) TS: anatomy

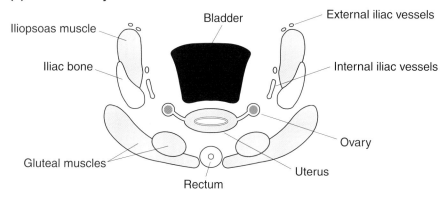

(iii) Ovary

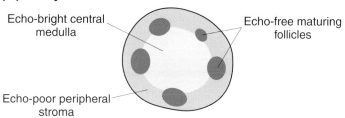

- The ovaries are attached to the uterus via the ovarian ligaments and a mobile mesovarium. As a result, they can be difficult to locate.

(iv) Uterine and ovarian cyclical change

	Uterine	*Ovarian*
Days 1–4: menstruation	Blood in cavity may cause separation of echo-bright endometrial lines	Small follicles (<5 mm)
Days 5–12: proliferation	Thin line of echo-bright endometrium thickens slowly	Dominant follicle enlarges (several follicles enlarge but one becomes dominant) — Dominant follicle
Days 13–16: peri-ovulatory	Endometrium appears echo-poor with echo-bright rim and central stripe: 'triple-line sign'	Dominant follicle ruptures — Ruptured follicle
Days 17–28: secretory	Thick irregular echo-bright line	Corpus luteum appears and slowly regresses — Corpus luteum

PERFORMING THE TRANSABDOMINAL SCAN

- **Patient position**: Supine.
- **Preparation**: Full bladder.
- Document LMP and take a brief gynaecological history.
- **Probe**: Low-frequency (3–5 MHz) curvilinear.
- **Machine**: Select gynaecological preset mode. Use two focal zones for imaging ovaries. Use tissue harmonics if the SNR is poor or with obese patients.
- **Method**: Acquire more than just the representative images for each step if pathology is found.

Probe position	*Instructions*

1. LS: uterus/endometrium
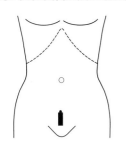
	- Begin by placing the probe midline in the suprapubic area.
	- Look for the bladder in LS with the uterus posterior to it. Tilt the probe (see below) and adjust the FOV to optimize the image. (*Hint*: Resting the end of the probe on the symphysis pubis gives good views.)
	- Now look for the endometrial stripe, which varies in appearance with both age and stage of the menstrual cycle:
	  – Is there any thickening or echotexture abnormalities?
	  – Measure its thickness
	- Acquire a representative image.

'Heel–toeing'

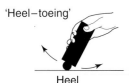

Heel Toe

Endometrial imaging

- Try to get the transducer parallel to the uterus for optimal imaging – by 'heel–toeing' the probe – e.g. if the uterus is anteverted/anteflexed then 'heel' the probe
- Always measure thickness in LS
- Do not include any cavity fluid in the measurement
- Normal values: <15 mm premenopausal; <5 mm postmenopausal

Probe position	*Instructions*
2. LS: lateral uterus 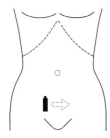	- Keep the probe in the LS position. - Scan out towards both adnexae by tilting the probe laterally and using the bladder as a window. While doing this, observe for any fibroids or echotexture abnormalities within the myometrium. - Acquire representative images of left and right lateral aspects of the uterus.

What to look for

Scan image

1.

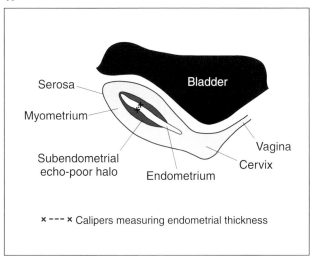

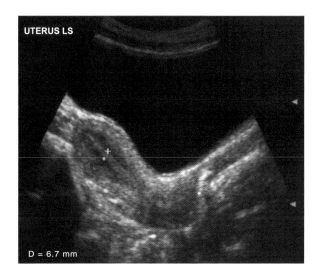

2.

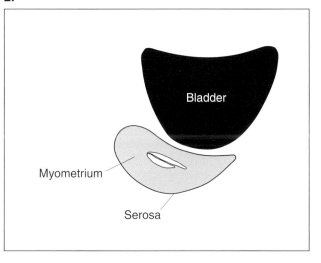

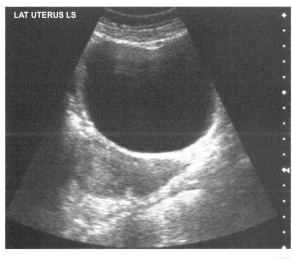

Probe position

3. LS: left and right adnexae

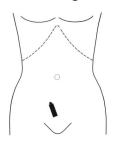

Instructions

- Scan out further laterally on both sides into each adnexal region.
- Look for each ovary in LS. Narrow the FOV, and use two focal zones. The internal iliac vessels are the lateral boundaries of the pelvis and useful landmarks to help locate the ovaries.
- If bowel gas is obscuring the image, try to displace it by pressing with your free hand.
- Are there any solid or cystic adnexal lesions?
- Acquire representative images of left and right adnexae, and the ovaries if identified.

Imaging the ovary

- Optimize image: narrow FOV, increase frequency, two focal zones, use zoom
- Is it an ovary?
- – Can echo-free follicles be seen?
- – Could it be bowel? (not round in both planes and displays peristalsis)
- After menopause, the ovaries atrophy and can be hard to see. In these cases, the aim of the study is simply to exclude any adnexal masses

---

What to look for

3a.

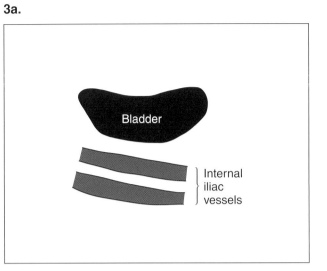

Scan image

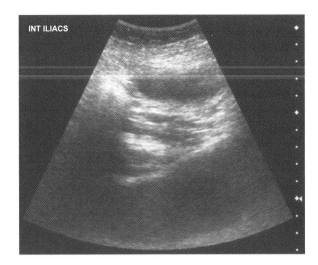

3b.

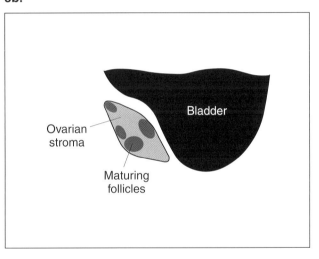

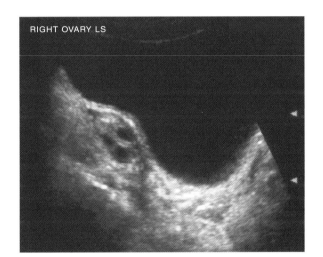

Probe position

4. TS: uterus

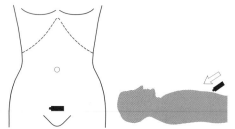

Instructions

- Now turn the probe 90° anticlockwise. Look for the TS image of the bladder with the uterus/vagina posterior to it.
- Adjust the FOV and focus position.
- Scan through the uterus from vagina to fundus by tilting the probe superiorly and inferiorly.
- Acquire representative images (e.g. of fundus/body/cervix).

5. TS: left and right adnexae

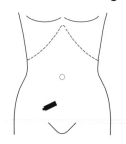

- Scan out into each adnexa by tilting the probe laterally and using the bladder as a window.
- Look for each ovary in TS. Narrow the FOV, and use two focal zones. The widest portion of the uterine body is a useful landmark to help locate the ovaries.
- Acquire representative images of left and right adnexae, and the ovaries if identified.

Complete the scan by imaging both kidneys as per Chapter 4 (looking for hydronephrosis from malignant ureteric obstruction)

What to look for

Scan image

4.

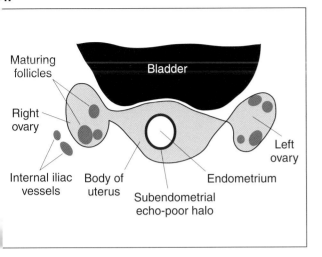

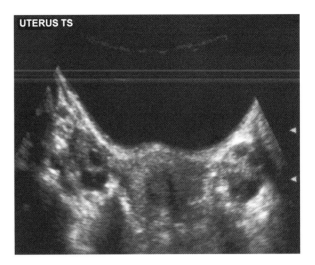

UTERUS TS

5.

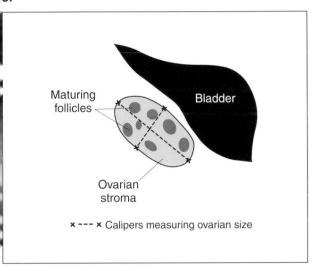

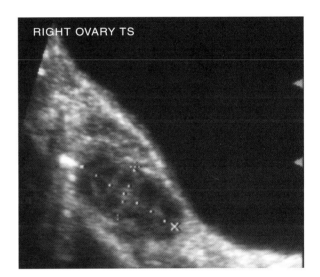

RIGHT OVARY TS

TRANSVAGINAL (TV) ANATOMY

(i) LS

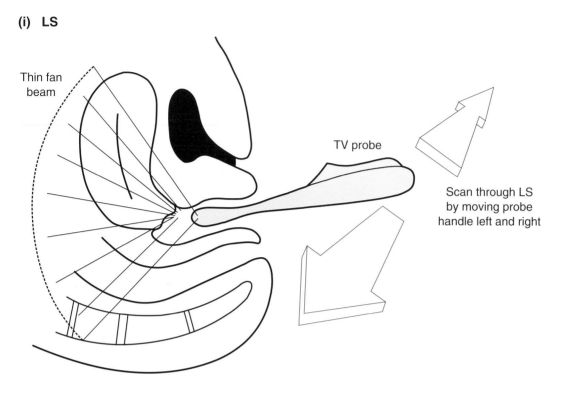

Thin fan beam

TV probe

Scan through LS by moving probe handle left and right

**Turn from LS into TS via 90°
anticlockwise handle rotation**

ii) TS

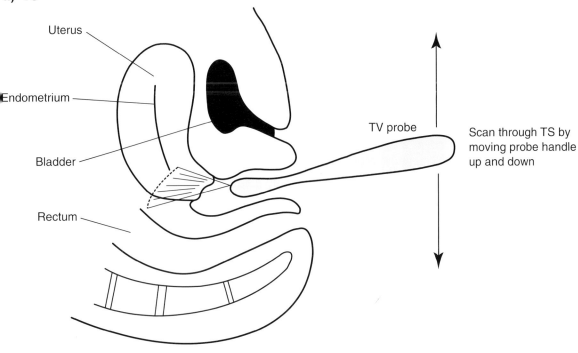

These are the two basic imaging planes employed in TV scanning. Remember that the fan beam is thin and that to scan through structures, the operator needs to move the probe in LS, TS and oblique planes.

PERFORMING THE TRANSVAGINAL SCAN

- It is advised that a chaperone be present during the examination. Explain the nature of the examination, asking for verbal consent.
- **Patient position**: Supine with legs abducted, knees flexed, and pad under buttocks or with buttocks at end of couch and feet supported on a chair.
- **Preparation**: Empty bladder.
- Document LMP and take a brief gynaecological history. Always ask if any area in the pelvis is particularly tender.
- **Probe**: Select TV probe and apply probe cover with gel.
- **Machine**: Select TV gynaecological preset mode. Use two focal zones for imaging the ovaries.
- **Method**: Acquire more than just the representative images for each step if pathology is found.

Probe position

1. LS: uterus/endometrium

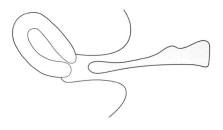

Instructions

- Begin by inserting the TV probe until resistance is felt.
- Look for the uterus LS. The probe/cervix interface will be at the top of the screen, with the fan beam coming down. An anteverted uterus appears on the left side of the screen and a retroverted uterus on the right.
- Now look for the endometrial stripe, which varies in appearance with both age and stage of the menstrual cycle:
  - Is there any thickening or echotexture abnormality?
  - Measure its thickness.
- Acquire a representative image.

2. LS: lateral uterus

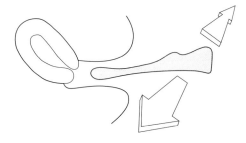

- Keep the probe in the LS position.
- Scan out through the body of the uterus towards both adnexae in the LS plane, by tilting the probe handle to the left and right. While doing this, observe for any fibroids or echotexture abnormalities within the myometrium.
- Acquire representative images of left and right lateral aspects of the uterus.

3. LS: left and right adnexae

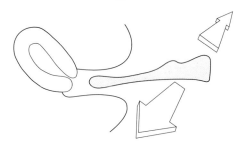

- Tilt the probe handle more laterally now into each adnexal region.
- Look for each ovary in LS. Narrow the FOV, and use two focal zones. The internal iliac vessels are the lateral boundaries of the pelvis, and are useful landmarks to help locate the ovaries.
- If bowel gas shadows interfere try displacing it by pressing with your free hand.
- Are there any solid or cystic adnexal lesions?
- Acquire representative images of left and right adnexae, and the ovaries if identified.

What to look for

Scan image

1.

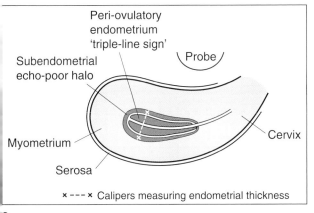

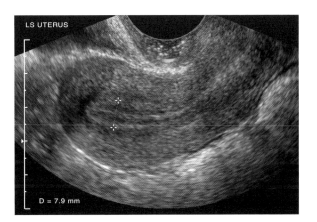

2.

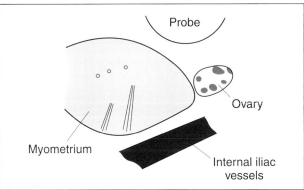

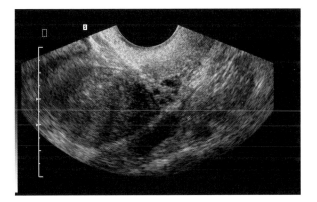

3.

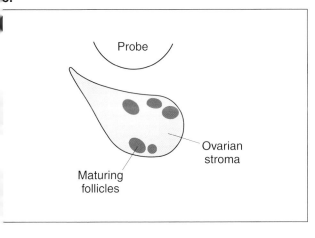

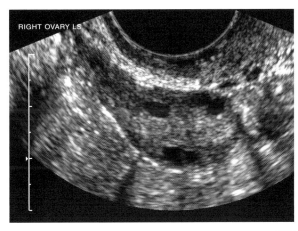

Probe position	**Instructions**

Probe position

4. TS: uterus

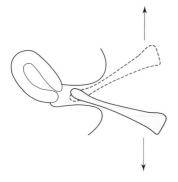

Instructions

- Now turn the probe handle 90° anticlockwise (withdraw it slightly first to avoid catching the cervix).
- Look for a TS image of the uterus.
- Adjust the FOV and focus position.
- Scan through the uterus from cervix to fundus. For an anteverted uterus, tilting the probe handle down (tip pointing up) will show the fundus. Tilt the tip down to look for the cervix.
  Hint: If the bed restricts the full range of probe movement, ask the patient to tilt the pelvis up.
- Acquire representative images (e.g. of fundus/body/cervix).

5. TS: left and right adnexae

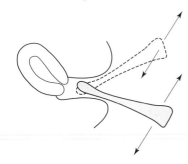

- Scan out into each adnexa by tilting the probe handle contralaterally.
- Look for each ovary in TS. Narrow the FOV, and use two focal zones. The widest portion of the uterine body is a useful landmark to help locate the ovaries.
- Acquire representative images of left and right adnexae, and the ovaries if identified.

Visceral slide assessment

The pelvic organs should normally move freely over each other on deep respiration and manual palpation (i.e. between hand and probe). If this does not occur, it may indicate inflammatory or malignant pathology.

Query: Polycystic ovarian syndrome (PCOS)?

- It is necessary to measure the ovarian volumes (a TV scan gives more accuracy than a TA scan).
- Calculate from LS and TS images, measuring the diameter in three planes. The split screen function can be helpful for this.
- Use the measurement package to calculate the volume (on most machines).
- Normal volume <10 cm^3 in premenopausal women.
- See the pathology section for more on this.

What to look for

4.

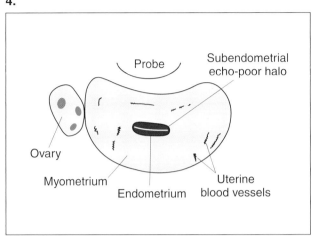

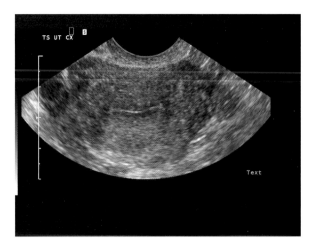

5.

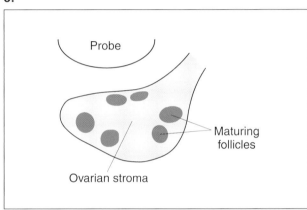

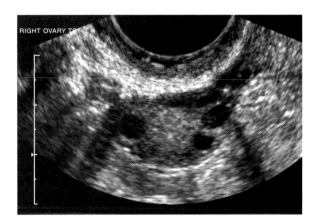

Measurement of ovary

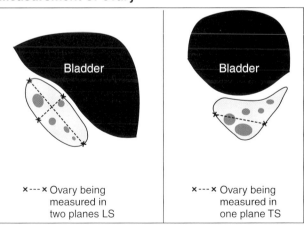

×---× Ovary being measured in two planes LS

×---× Ovary being measured in one plane TS

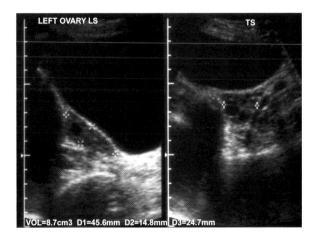

PATHOLOGY

1. Uterine fibroids (leiomyoma)

These are a very common finding (25% of premenopausal women). Fibroids are benign smooth muscle tumours with a fibrous element. They are oestrogen-dependent: they can grow rapidly during pregnancy, and tend to regress after the menopause. They are often asymptomatic, but can cause menorrhagia, pain or subfertility, depending on their size and location:

- mural: arise within the myometrium (95% of fibroids)
- submucosal: protrude into the endometrial cavity
- subserosal: project from the uterine surface

Ultrasound features

- Focal uterine enlargement
- Well-defined echo-poor mass with characteristic lamellated/whirled internal echo pattern
- May contain echo-bright areas of calcification or degeneration
- Can also occur as a diffuse uterine process

2. Nabothian cysts

These are small benign inclusion cysts, which are commonly seen in the region of the endocervical canal. They are of no clinical significance.

Ultrasound features
- Smooth edge
- Thin wall
- Echo-free contents
- Postacoustic enhancement

3. Polycystic ovarian syndrome (PCOS)

PCOS is diagnosed on the basis of clinical, biochemical and ultrasound findings. Only about 50% of PCOS patients will have the typical ultrasound findings. The absence of these therefore does not preclude the diagnosis.

Ultrasound features
- Ovarian volume >10 cm^3
- >10 follicles in an ovary in any one imaging plane
- Peripheral ovarian stroma is echo-bright
- Peripheral ovarian stroma is of increased volume

Hint: PCOS is not to be confused with multicystic ovaries, which are seen at the menarche and in anorexia (normal ovarian volumes, less numerous larger follicles!).

What to look for

Scan image

1. Uterine fibroid

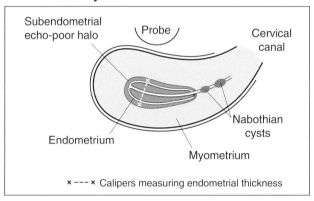

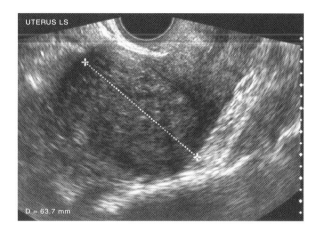

2. Nabothian cysts

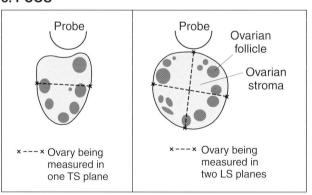

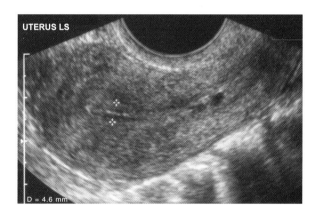

3. PCOS

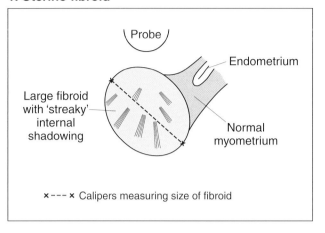

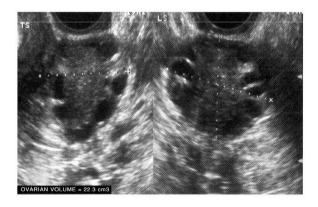

4. Ovarian cysts

When an ovarian lesion is identified, it is important to classify its appearance as benign, suspicious or malignant. This will determine if follow-up is required.

(a) Benign

- These display the typical features of a simple cyst (see previous pages).
- They measure <3 cm in a premenopausal woman; <5 cm in a postmenopausal woman. They are usually physiological (e.g. follicular cysts). They are very common and of no clinical significance. They do not need to be followed up.

(b) Suspicious

These are cysts that have a slightly more complex appearance, often caused by internal haemorrhage (e.g. corpus luteal cyst). Suspicious features include:

- large size: >3 cm in a premenopausal woman; >5 cm in a postmenopausal woman
- internal echoes
- fine internal septations

A follow-up scan is needed in 6–8 weeks (to check for size reduction/resolution).

(c) Malignant

These cystic lesions have a frankly neoplastic appearance. They are usually due to primary ovarian cancer. Features suggestive of malignancy include:

- thick irregular walls
- thick internal septations
- internal echoes
- papillary nodules on cyst wall
- usually >5 cm

Look for other malignant features:

- hydronephrosis
- liver metastases
- omental cake
- ascites
- pleural effusions
- peritoneal deposits

Check the patient's CA-125 (blood marker of ovarian cancer). Refer for further imaging (e.g. MRI).

What to look for

4a. Simple ovarian cyst

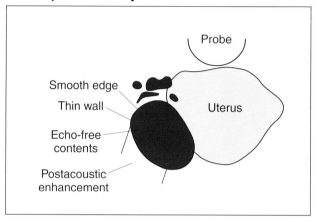

4b. Complex ovarian cyst

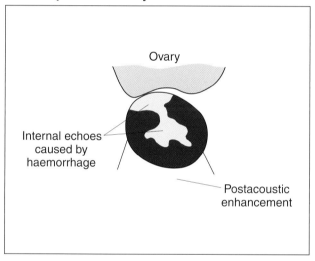

4c. Ovarian malignancy

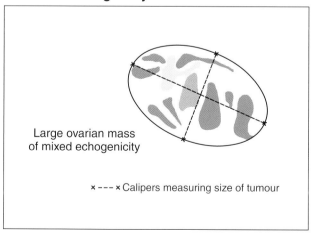

Scan image

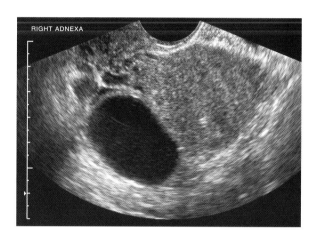

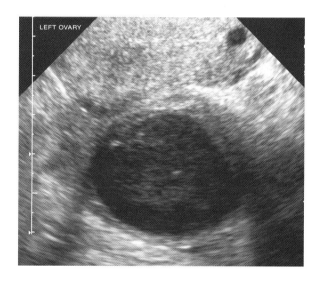

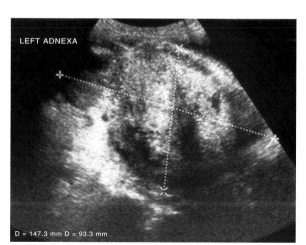

5. Endometrial thickening

The endometrium is considered thickened on ultrasound if:

- >15 mm in a premenopausal woman
- >5 mm in a postmenopausal woman

(a) Focal thickening

This can be caused by an endometrial polyp or submucosal fibroid.

(b) Diffuse thickening

- Endometrial hyperplasia:
  - physiological
  - drug-induced (tamoxifen, HRT)
  - oestrogen-secreting tumours
- Endometrial carcinoma:
  - this can arise from hyperplasia or occur de novo
  - it is a common malignancy in postmenopausal women

Ultrasound cannot reliably distinguish between hyperplasia and carcinoma, so hysteroscopy and biopsy are required in all cases.

(c) Features suspicious of malignancy

- Thickened endometrium with irregular margin
- Endometrial mass of mixed echogenicity
- Endometrial mass seen to be infiltrating into the myometrium
- Extrauterine deposits

What to look for

5a. Focal thickening

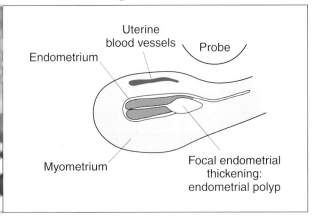

5b. Diffuse thickening

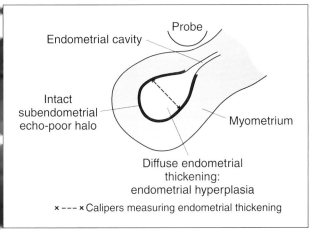

5c. Malignant thickening

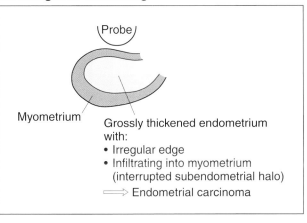

Scan image

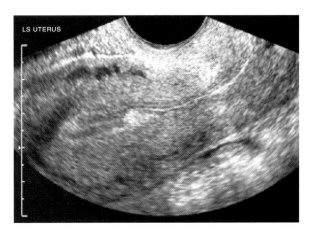

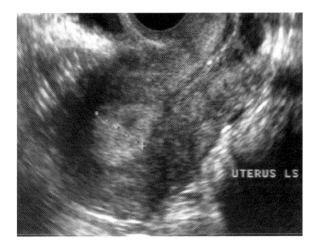

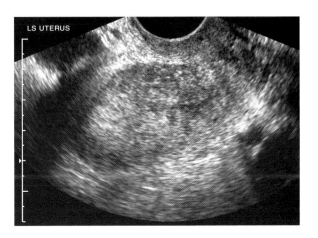

6. Intrauterine contraceptive device (IUCD)

Some coils can be harder to see than others, and it may only be possible to see their endpoints. To be effective, they must be positioned <5 mm from the upper end of the endometrium.

Ultrasound features

- Usually identified as a hyperechoic structure within the cavity
- Casts a strong acoustic shadow

7. False pelvic mass

A mirror-image artefact of the bladder is seen posterior to the uterus. It can easily be mistaken for a pelvic mass. It is caused by reflection of the beam from bowel loops in the pouch of Douglas.

Ultrasound features

- Lack of well-defined superior and inferior walls of the 'mass'
- The 'mass' is located too far posteriorly to be anatomically possible

In slim patients, beware the sacrum!

What to look for

6. IUCD

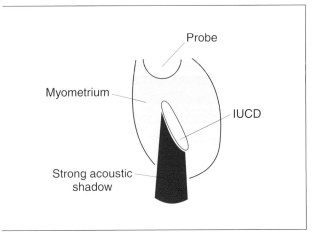

7. False pelvic mass

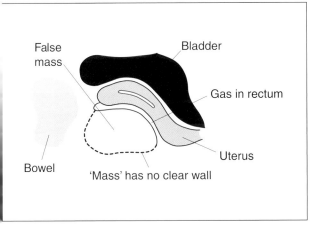

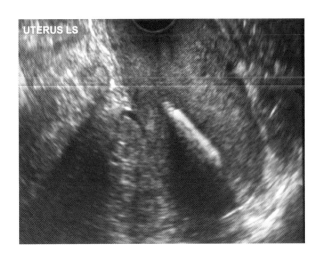

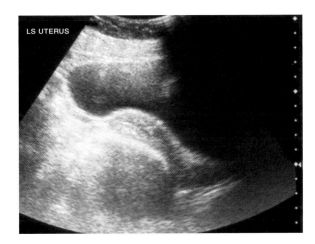

11
<u>Early pregnancy</u>

USEFUL ANATOMY

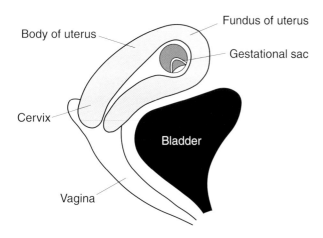

5¹/₂ weeks' gestation

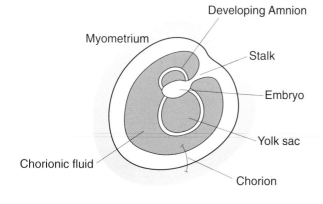

Later

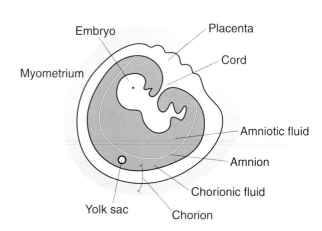

Key points

- 80% of women have an anteverted or anteflexed uterus.
- The gestational sac is usually sited in the fundal region of the uterus.
- The yolk sac is normally the first structure to be seen within the gestational sac. Its presence confirms that this is a gestation and not just a fluid collection.

PERFORMING THE SCAN

The primary role of ultrasound in the first trimester of pregnancy is to confirm the presence of a live intrauterine pregnancy and to distinguish this from a pregnancy failure or ectopic pregnancy.

Appropriate medical and nursing support must be available, and there should be access to a quiet side room when bad news is given. Allow partners to be present during the scan. It is advised that a chaperone should always be present (essential for male examiners). Begin by explaining the nature of the examination and the reasons for doing it, asking the patient for verbal consent. Take a brief obstetric history, and document dates of the LMP and pregnancy test.

The scan can be performed either transabdominally or transvaginally.

Transabdominal scan

Patient position: Supine.

Preparation: In thin patients, a full bladder is not always needed. Provided that the uterus is anteverted, good visualization of its contents can usually be achieved.

Probe: Low-frequency (3–5 MHz) curvilinear.

Machine: Select early pregnancy or obstetric preset mode, and use two focal zones. Use tissue harmonics if the SNR is poor or with obese patients.

Transvaginal scan

Patient position: Supine with legs abducted (see Chapter 10).

Preparation: Empty bladder.

Probe: Select TV probe and apply probe cover with gel.

Machine: Select early pregnancy or gynaecological preset mode, and use two focal zones.

The scanning techniques are basically the same as those used in a regular gynaecological scan. Reference should be made to Chapter 10.

Safe practice

- The mechanical index (MI) should be kept to the lowest level that still allows an image to be achieved: it is recommended that an MI $\leqslant$ 0.7 be used.

  Minimize exposure of the fetus by using the freeze and ciné loop functions to reduce the scan time.

- Colour and/or spectral Doppler of the fetus should usually be avoided in the first trimester.

Early-pregnancy reporting

The report should normally include the following information:

- Gestational sac position: is it intrauterine?
- Fetal number.
- If the pregnancy is multifetal, indicate the number of placentae (chorionicity).
- Fetal heart pulsation: present/absent?
- Mean sac diameter (MSD) or if present, CRL/BPD.
- Estimated gestational age and which measurement was used for this.
- If no embryo is seen, the presence or absence of the yolk sac should be indicated.
- Include a description of any gynaecological masses that are present.

Several terms are used to conclude the report of a pregnancy failure. These include missed abortion, missed miscarriage and failed pregnancy. Many also use 'missed miss' to cover everything, including anembryonic pregnancy. It is recommended that each department agree on a common terminology.

Probe position

1. LS: uterus/gestational sac

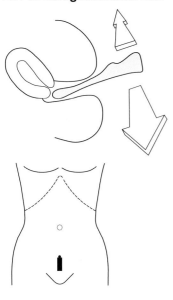

Instructions

- For either TA or TV method, begin by imaging the uterus in the LS plane. Initially use the widest FOV. Adjust the depth and focus position (for more details, see Chapter 10).
- Look for an intrauterine gestational sac, and if present, observe:
  - if it contains a visible yolk sac or embryo(s)
  - if any heart pulsations can be seen
  - the relationship of the sac to the cervix

  It may help to narrow the FOV and use zoom
- Acquire a representative image.

Fetal heart pulsation

- This should definitely be visible when the crown–rump length is measured as >6 mm via a TV scan or >10 mm via TA.
- Heart pulsations may be detected with crown–rump lengths as low as 3 mm.

Time-motion (M-mode)

- Now formally assess for a fetal heart pulsation in real time:
  - select M-mode function
  - on most machines, a dual image will appear (a real-time image and an M-mode image)
  - place the M-mode line across the estimated position of the fetal chest
  - look for M-mode evidence of heart pulsation
- Acquire a representative image.
- Now measure:
  - gestational sac size
  - crown–rump length and/or
  - biparietal diameter (see below for more details)
- Acquire representative images.

What to look for

Scan image

1a. LS: uterus TA

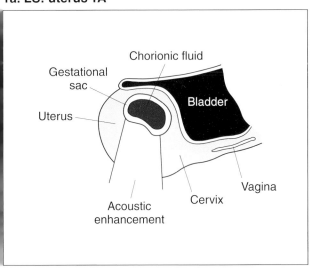

Chorionic fluid

Gestational sac

Bladder

Uterus

Vagina

Acoustic enhancement

Cervix

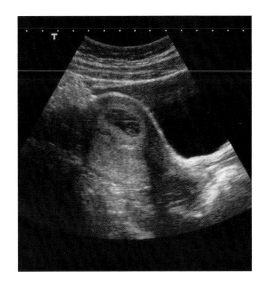

1b. LS: uterus TV

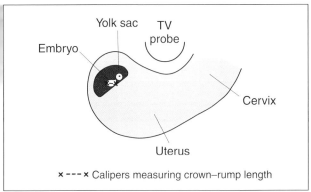

Yolk sac

TV probe

Embryo

Cervix

Uterus

x‐‐‐x Calipers measuring crown–rump length

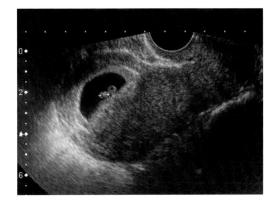

1c. TS: time–motion mode

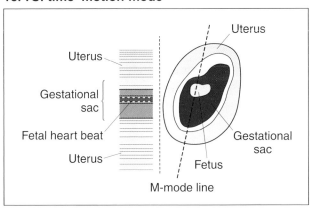

Uterus

Uterus

Gestational sac

Fetal heart beat

Uterus

Gestational sac

Fetus

M-mode line

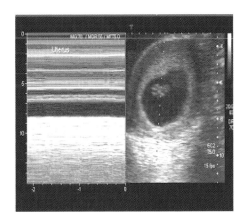

Probe position	Instructions

2. TS: uterus/gestational sac
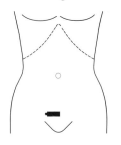
	• Now image the uterus in the TS plane via a 90° anticlockwise probe rotation for both TV and TA methods (for more details, see Chapter 10).
	• Scan through the uterus from cervix to fundus:
	  – again looking for an intrauterine gestational sac
	  – when doing this, remember to check for any fibroids or echotexture abnormalities within the myometrium
	• Acquire a representative image.

3. LS/TS: left and right adnexae 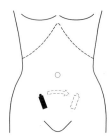	• When performing a pregnancy scan, it is good practice to also examine the ovaries and adnexal regions for pathology. • Scan out towards both adnexae in the LS and TS planes by angling the probe laterally for both TV and TA methods (for more details, see Chapter 10). • In particular, look for any signs to suggest an ectopic pregnancy (see pathology section). • Acquire representative images of left and right adnexae, and the ovaries if identified.

ESTIMATING GESTATIONAL AGE

There are several ways in which this can be done, and three commonly used methods are discussed below. Note that using a TV scanning method will permit more accurate estimations.

1. Gestational sac size

• If a gestational sac is detected, the mean sac diameter (MSD) can be used to estimate the gestational age of the embryo.
• Calculate the MSD using one LS and one TS image and measuring the sac diameter in three planes. The split screen function can be helpful for this.
• Add all three measurements together and divide by 3: this is the MSD (measured in millimetres)
• Acquire a representative image.
• By cross-reference with special charts, the MSD can be used to estimate the gestational age of the embryo.

What to look for

Scan image

2. TS: uterus

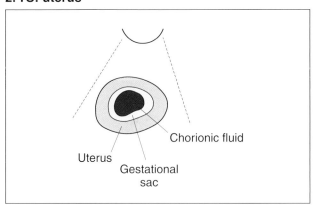

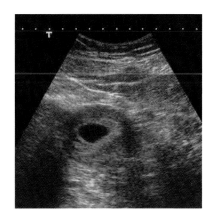

3. TS: adnexae

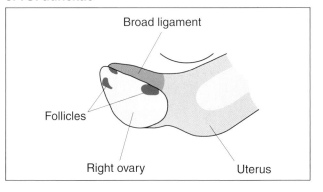

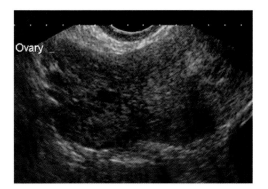

1. Measurement: gestational sac

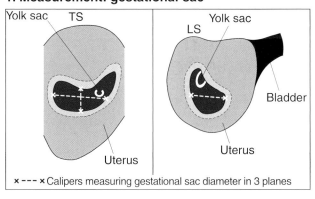

× - - - × Calipers measuring gestational sac diameter in 3 planes

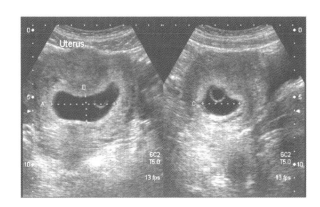

2. Crown–rump length (CRL)

- If an embryo is detected within the gestational sac, its CRL should be used to estimate gestational age.
- First optimize the image for accuracy of measurement: narrow the FOV, use multiple focal zones and use the zoom function.
- The embryo should be measured in its longest axis, which is found by gentle probe rotation in LS, TS and oblique planes.
- When found, freeze the image.
- Select the CRL measurement package (on most machines).
- Place one caliper at the upper end of the embryo (its crown) and another at the lower end (its rump).
- The machine will display an estimated gestational age (if this function is not available, the distance can be cross-referenced with a special CRL chart).

Hint: Primitive rhomboencephalon can make the head look like a yolk sac. Common mistakes include omitting the head or including the yolk sac in the measurement!

3. Biparietal diameter (BPD)

- If an embryo's gestational age has been estimated at 13 weeks or more by CRL then BPD should be used to give a more accurate estimation.
- First optimize the image: narrow the FOV, use multiple focal zones and use the zoom function.
- For standardized, reproducible results, the head should be measured in a true axial (TS) plane.
  Find this via fine manipulation of the probe, looking for the following key anatomical landmarks:
  - 'rugby ball'-shaped head
  - interhemispheric fissure (IHF)
  - equal hemisphere diameters
  - thalamus
  - cavum septum pellucidum
  - anterior horns of the lateral ventricles
- Select the BPD measurement package (on most machines).
- Measure from outer to inner skull table at 90° to the IHF.
- The machine will display an estimated gestational age (if this function is not available, the distance can be cross-referenced with a special BPD chart).

What to look for

2a. Measurement: CRL

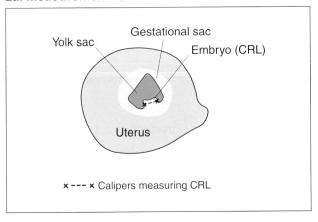

2b. Measurement: CRL

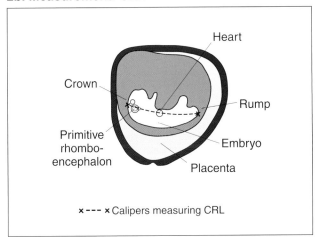

3. Measurement: fetal head

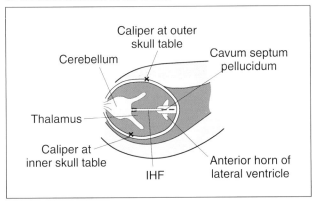

Scan image

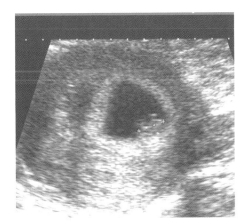

CRL 13 mm = 8 weeks

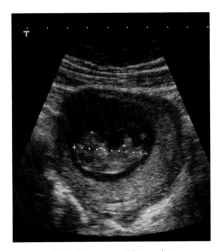

CRL 36 mm = 10 weeks

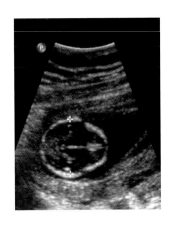

EARLY PREGNANCY ABNORMALITIES

1. Multifetal pregnancy

- State the presence/absence and thickness of the septum.
- Assess the number of placentae (chorionicity): look for the lambda sign (placental tissue forming in the septum between the embryos).
- Assess the number of amniotic cavities (amnionicity).
- Indicate on the report whether the pregnancy is monochorionic/monoamniotic, monochorionic/diamniotic or dichorionic/diamniotic.
- Note the relative position of the fetuses.
- If possible, assess whether the fetuses are of the same sex.
- A diagram of the fetuses on the report is helpful and will assist in subsequent scans.

2. Corpus luteal cyst of pregnancy

Following fertilisation the corpus luteum persists (due to β-HCG). In this condition bleeding occurs into it, often causing pain. Most resolve spontaneously.

Ultrasound features

- Most are <5 cm in size
- Thin wall
- Display internal echoes from the blood
- This complex appearance can mimic an ovarian malignancy; if there is any doubt, repeat the scan in 6–8 weeks time (see Chapter 10 for more on ovarian cysts)

3. Subchorionic haemorrhage

This is venous bleeding into the subchorionic space extending to the margin of the placenta. It usually occurs in early pregnancy and is associated with smoking. It has a favourable prognosis.

Ultrasound features

- The marginal edge of the placenta is separated from the myometrium
- If the bleed is recent, it may contain internal echoes – old bleeds are echo-free

Hint: Large retroplacental haemorrhage (abruption) tends to occur in late pregnancy and has a poor outcome. It is not reliably diagnosed by ultrasound.

What to look for

1. Dichorionic pregnancy: lambda sign

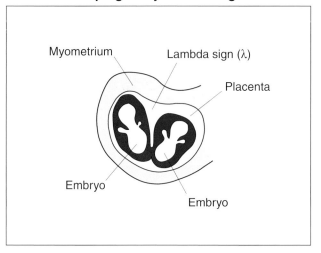

Myometrium

Lambda sign (λ)

Placenta

Embryo

Embryo

2. Corpus luteum of pregnancy

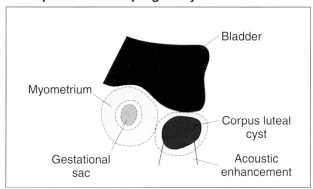

Bladder

Myometrium

Corpus luteal cyst

Gestational sac

Acoustic enhancement

3. Subchorionic haemorrhage

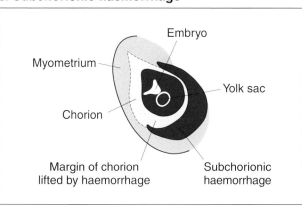

Embryo

Myometrium

Yolk sac

Chorion

Margin of chorion lifted by haemorrhage

Subchorionic haemorrhage

Scan image

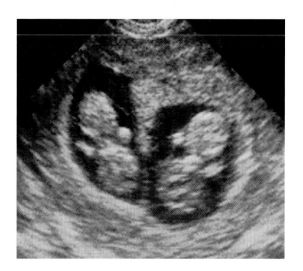

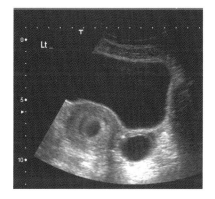

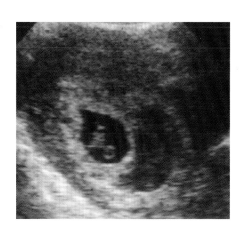

4. Incomplete abortion/retained products of conception (RPOC)

This is when fetal death occurs and some placental/fetal tissue remains within the endometrial cavity, usually causing heavy bleeding.

Do not always assume that debris in the endometrial cavity is due to RPOC. Relate the findings to any prior scans. If the patient has previously been shown to have had an intrauterine gestational sac/embryo then the diagnosis can be made confidently. Otherwise:

- If the β-hCG level is falling then the report should indicate that RPOC is the most likely cause
- If the β-hCG level is unknown then an ectopic pregnancy with an associated decidual reaction cannot be excluded

Ultrasound features

- Echo-bright or heterogeneous material is seen within the endometrial cavity

5. Hydatidiform mole

This rare but important condition occurs in early pregnancy and is caused by trophoblastic tissue in the placenta undergoing excessive proliferation. Occasionally, fetal tissue forms, but this is non-viable. Patients present with first-trimester bleeding and hyperemesis caused by very elevated β-hCG levels.

Treatment involves referral to a specialist centre for evacuation of uterine contents and serial monitoring of β-hCG levels to ensure complete regression. Approximately 10% will develop an invasive mole or malignant choriocarcinoma (persistently elevated β-hCG levels) and the treatment is with chemotherapy. The prognosis is generally good.

Ultrasound features

- In the early stages, the uterus is enlarged and filled with echo-bright material: 'snowstorm' appearance
- As the mole progresses, easily visible echo-poor cystic spaces develop within it: 'bunch of grapes' appearance
- Associated with large ovarian theca-lutein cysts (due to excessive β-hCG stimulation)

What to look for

4. RPOC

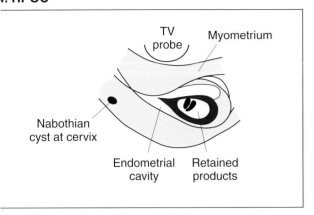

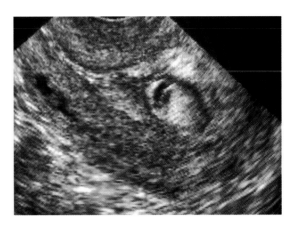

5. Hydatidiform mole

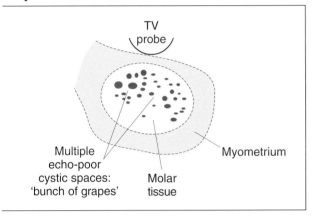

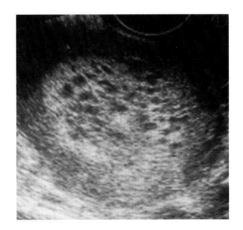

6. Embryonic demise

The following are signs of fetal death:

6a. Empty sac sign

- A gestational sac, MSD >20 mm (TA or TV) with no visible yolk sac
- A gestational sac, MSD >25 mm (TA or TV) with no visible embryo

Causes of an empty sac:
- missed abortion
- anembryonic pregnancy
- pseudogestational sac from an ectopic pregnancy

6b. Empty-amnion sign

- An amnion is clearly visible without the presence of an embryo

6c. Absent fetal heart pulsation

- Embryo with a CRL >10 mm, TA with no detectable heart pulsation
- Embryo with a CRL >6 mm, TV with no detectable heart pulsation
- Flat M-mode trace

Safe diagnosis requires the independent observation of two qualified ultrasound practitioners. If either of the practitioners is in doubt, a rescan in 7–10 days is required. If a second practitioner is not available, the patient should be informed of the first practitioner's findings and offered the choice of proceeding to management or waiting for a second opinion on another day.

6d. Failure of interval growth

- Allowing for interobserver variation, a failed pregnancy can be confirmed if there has been no growth of the MSD after a 1-week interval

What to look for

6. Embryonic demise

6a. Empty sac

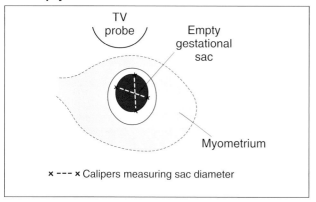

6b. Empty-amnion sign

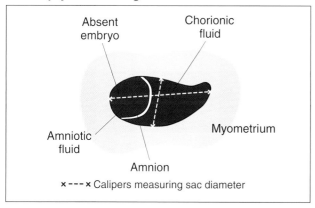

6c. Absent fetal heart pulsation

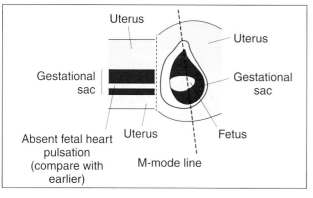

Scan image

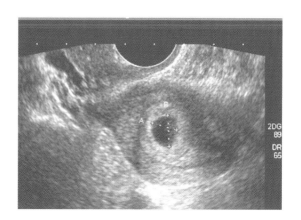

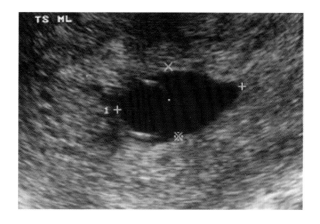

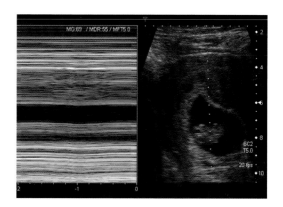

7. Ectopic pregnancy

This is implantation of a pregnancy outside the endometrial cavity.

- The incidence is 0.3–1.6% of all pregnancies and accounts for 10% of maternal deaths.
- If the patient is collapsed, ultrasound is not appropriate. Do not delay operative treatment.
- Referrals for ectopic pregnancy should have both TA and TV scans unless the diagnosis is clear from the TA scan.
- The role of ultrasound is to attempt to localize the pregnancy.
- If an intrauterine pregnancy is found, an ectopic pregnancy is virtually excluded because the combination of intrauterine and ectopic pregnancy is extremely rare in normal conceptions (1 in 30 000).
- In stimulated in vitro fertilization (IVF) pregnancies, the heterotopic pregnancy rate is much higher.
- Beware a pseudogestational sac caused by decidual reaction.
- The ultrasound findings must be correlated with the clinical symptoms and β-hCG levels:
  - An empty uterus and a positive pregnancy test can be due to an intrauterine pregnancy less than 5 weeks, a miscarriage or an ectopic pregnancy.
  - It is better to use a discriminatory value for β-hCG > 1000 IU, at which level an embryo should always be visible. Serial β-hCG testing is useful in equivocal cases.

Ultrasound features

- Demonstration of an extrauterine embryonic heartbeat is diagnostic, but this is not a common finding
- The presence of free fluid containing echoes (haemoperitoneum) has a strong positive predictive value (best seen using TV method)
- Echo-bright endometrial thickening from hormonal stimulation by the ectopic is common; a pseudogestational sac is seen in 20%
- A solid/cystic adnexal mass may be seen. This often has a concentric appearance to it, and has been likened to a 'doughnut'
- In reality, it can be difficult to distinguish these adnexal masses from other pathology, e.g. complex ovarian lesions (see the pathology section in Chapter 10)

A normal TV scan does not exclude an ectopic pregnancy

Hint: The use of colour Doppler for detecting peritrophoblastic blood flow has been shown to have no benefit over greyscale ultrasound in the diagnosis of ectopic pregnancy.

What to look for

Scan image

7a. Ectopic pregnancy: haemoperitoneum

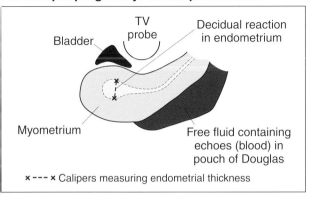

- TV probe
- Bladder
- Decidual reaction in endometrium
- Myometrium
- Free fluid containing echoes (blood) in pouch of Douglas
- ×---× Calipers measuring endometrial thickness

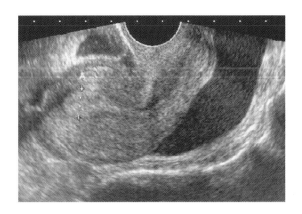

7b. Ectopic pregnancy: adnexal mass

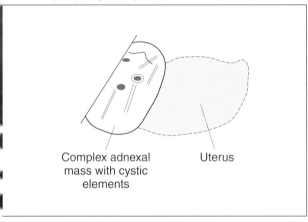

- Complex adnexal mass with cystic elements
- Uterus

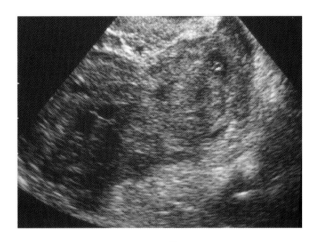

7c. Ectopic pregnancy: extrauterine gestational sac

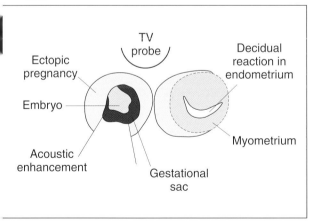

- TV probe
- Ectopic pregnancy
- Decidual reaction in endometrium
- Embryo
- Acoustic enhancement
- Gestational sac
- Myometrium

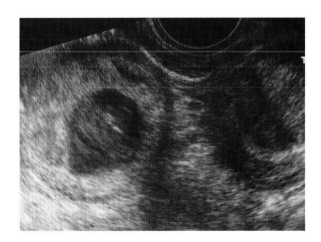

12
<u>Thyroid</u>

ANATOMY

Transverse section

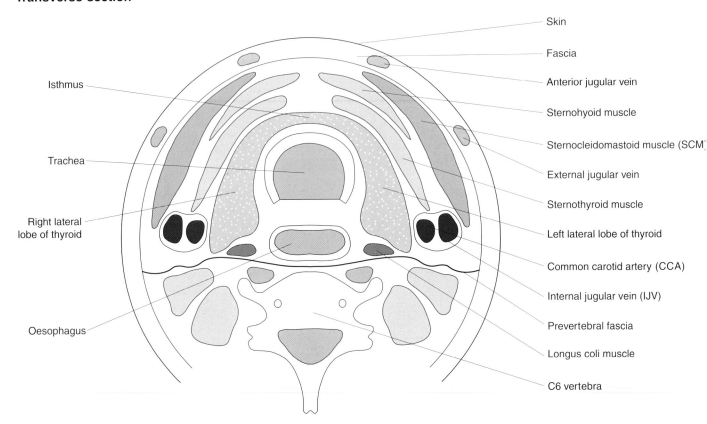

Isthmus

Trachea

Right lateral
lobe of thyroid

Oesophagus

Skin

Fascia

Anterior jugular vein

Sternohyoid muscle

Sternocleidomastoid muscle (SCM)

External jugular vein

Sternothyroid muscle

Left lateral lobe of thyroid

Common carotid artery (CCA)

Internal jugular vein (IJV)

Prevertebral fascia

Longus coli muscle

C6 vertebra

Anterior view

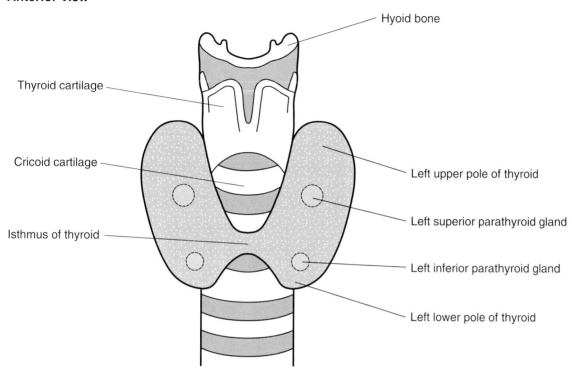

Hyoid bone

Thyroid cartilage

Cricoid cartilage

Left upper pole of thyroid

Left superior parathyroid gland

Isthmus of thyroid

Left inferior parathyroid gland

Left lower pole of thyroid

Key points

1. The thyroid gland has two lateral lobes and a midline isthmus.
2. The lateral lobes are often asymmetrical; the right tends to be more vascular and larger.
3. Each lobe has a superior and inferior pole.
4. The normal craniocaudal length of the thyroid gland is <4 cm.
5. There are four parathyroid glands lying posterior to the thyroid gland.
6. The normal craniocaudal length of each parathyroid gland is <6 mm.

Surface landmarks of thyroid

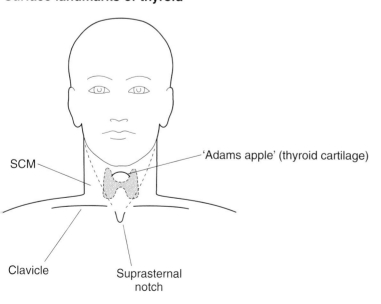

SCM

'Adams apple' (thyroid cartilage)

Clavicle

Suprasternal notch

PERFORMING THE SCAN

- **Patient position**: Supine with neck extended.
- **Preparation**: None.
- **Probe**: High-frequency (7.5 MHz) linear.
- **Machine**: Select 'small parts' preset on machine. Use tissue harmonics if the SNR is poor. Use at least two focal zones, with one positioned at the posterior aspect of the thyroid gland.
- **Method**: Do not apply any pressure to the probe, because this can be uncomfortable for the patient.

Probe position

1. TS

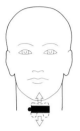
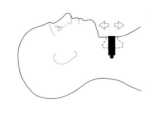

Instructions

- Place the probe just inferior to the thyroid cartilage.
- Scan through the thyroid in TS.
- The normal thyroid gland:
  - is more echogenic than the SCM
  - has a homogenous echotexture
  - is highly vascular
- Take note of the:
  - echogenicity
  - surface outline
  - texture
  - size
- Check for any:
  - calcification (micro or macro)
  - solid lesions (size, mass effect)
  - cysts
- Depending on the clinical history and ultrasound findings, turn on colour/power Doppler to assess for:
  - hyperaemia
  - neovascularization of any solid lesions
- Take representative image(s).

2. LS

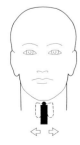
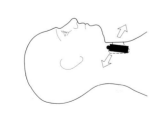

- Rotate the probe clockwise through 90°.
- Scan through the thyroid in LS.
- Observe the thyroid characteristics as described in Step 1.
- If the whole gland is not on the screen, it may be enlarged; measure the craniocaudal length to check for a goitre. If necessary, use a dual screen. The normal craniocaudal thyroid length is <4 cm.
- Take representative image(s).

What to look for

1.

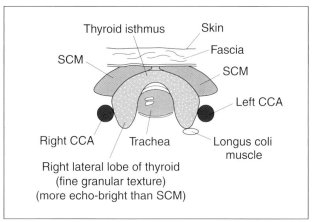

Scan image

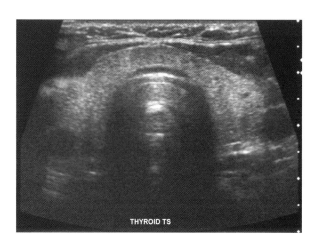

2.

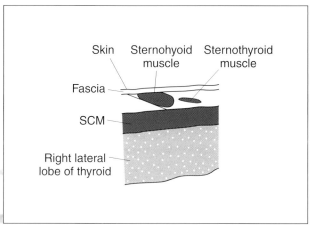

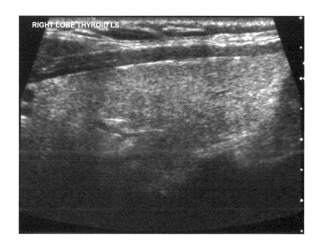

PATHOLOGY

1. Graves' disease

This is an autoimmune disease with a female-to-male ratio of 8:1, affecting ages 20–40 years. Usually associated with hyperthyroidism.

Ultrasound features

- Diffusely enlarged thyroid
- Homogenous, i.e. loss of fine granular echotexture
- Normal echogenicity or echo-bright
- Displays increased blood flow with colour/power Doppler

2. Hashimoto's thyroiditis

This is an autoimmune disease with a female-to-male ratio of 12:1, affecting ages 30–50 years. Usually hypothyroid.

Ultrasound features

- Diffusely enlarged thyroid
- Heterogenous, with coarse echotexture
- Echo-poor

3. Multinodular goitre

This has a female-to-male ratio of 3:1, and in the age range 50–70 years. Usually normal thyroid function.

Ultrasound features

- Irregular enlarged thyroid
- Heterogenous with multiple nodules
- Nodules can be solid, cystic or solid/cystic
- Nodules >7 mm

What to look for

1. Graves' disease

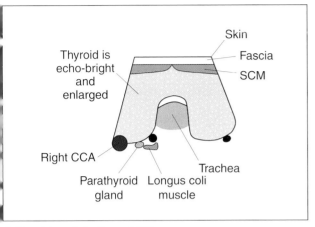

- Skin
- Fascia
- SCM
- Thyroid is echo-bright and enlarged
- Right CCA
- Parathyroid gland
- Longus coli muscle
- Trachea

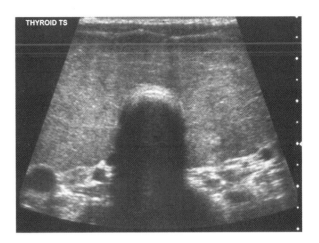

2. Hashimoto's thyroiditis

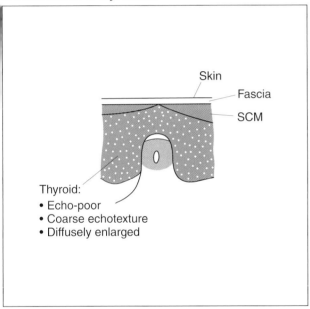

- Skin
- Fascia
- SCM
- Thyroid:
  - Echo-poor
  - Coarse echotexture
  - Diffusely enlarged

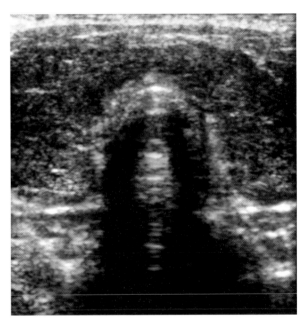

3. Multinodular goitre

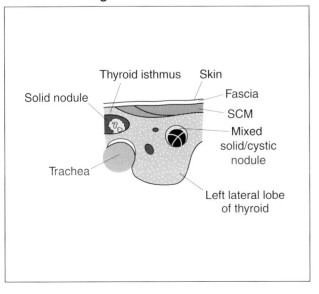

- Solid nodule
- Thyroid isthmus
- Skin
- Fascia
- SCM
- Mixed solid/cystic nodule
- Trachea
- Left lateral lobe of thyroid

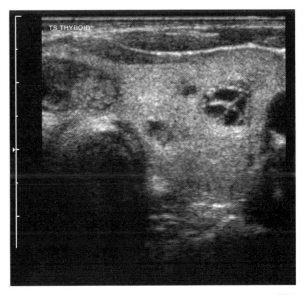

4. Thyroid carcinoma

There are five types: papillary, follicular, anaplastic, medullary and lymphoma. The female-to-male ratio is 3:1. Papillary and follicular types affect ages 20–40 years and anaplastic ages >60 years. Note that calcification is useful to determine whether a nodule is malignant or benign:

- microcalcification (<2 mm): high positive predictive value for malignancy
- macrocalcification (>2 mm): degeneration/postinflammatory, often rim calcifications

Ultrasound features

- Predominantly single, but may be multiple
- Mass usually >7 mm
- Solid or partially cystic
- Irregular margins
- Exert mass effect
- Echo-poor
- Microcalcification
- Hypervascular (with colour/power Doppler)

What to look for

Scan image

4a. Thyroid carcinoma

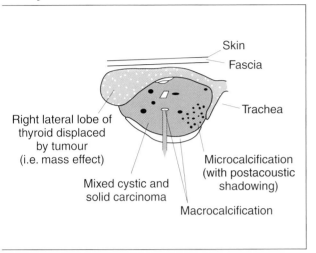

- Skin
- Fascia
- Trachea
- Right lateral lobe of thyroid displaced by tumour (i.e. mass effect)
- Microcalcification (with postacoustic shadowing)
- Mixed cystic and solid carcinoma
- Macrocalcification

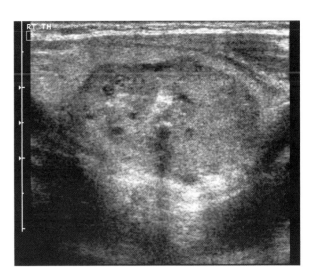

4b. Thyroid carcinoma

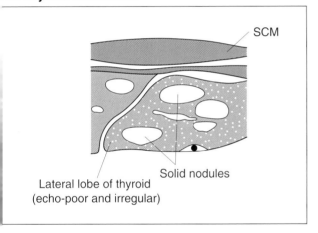

- SCM
- Solid nodules
- Lateral lobe of thyroid (echo-poor and irregular)

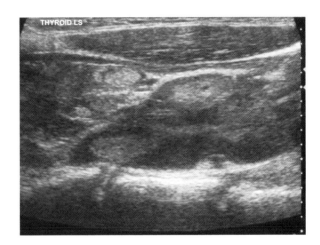

5. Enlarged parathyroid glands

Causes include adenoma, carcinoma and hyperplasia (e.g. in patients with longstanding chronic renal failure (CRF)).

Ultrasound features

- >6 mm
- More echo-poor than thyroid
- Hypervascular (with colour/power Doppler)
- Diffusely enlarged (with hyperplasia)
- Heterogenous (with adenoma or carcinoma)

Hint: Do not confuse the longus coli muscle with an enlarged parathyroid gland. Confirm that it is a parathyroid gland by scanning in TS and LS.

6. Cervical lymphadenopathy

Causes include infection, metastases and lymphoma.

Ultrasound features of reactive nodes

- Elliptical
- Long axis <10 mm, short axis <7 mm
- Echo-bright hilum of fat
- Echo-poor cortex

Ultrasound features of pathological nodes

- Spherical
- >10 mm long axis
- Loss of echo-bright hilum
- May exert a mass effect on surrounding structures

What to look for

5. Enlarged parathyroid gland

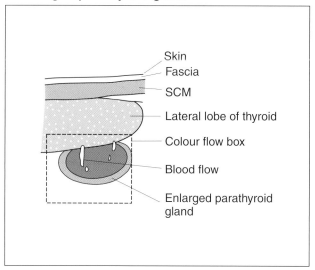

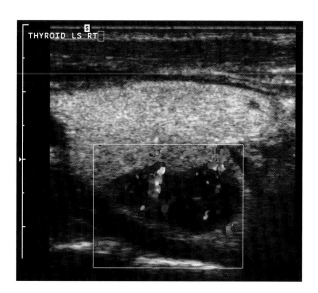

6. Cervical lymphadenopathy

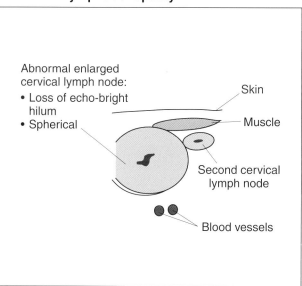

Abnormal enlarged cervical lymph node:
- Loss of echo-bright hilum
- Spherical

Skin

Muscle

Second cervical lymph node

Blood vessels

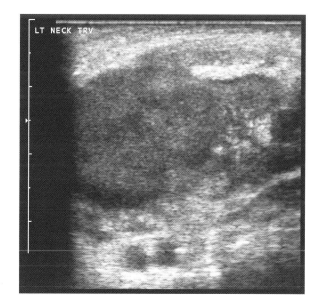

Index